Handbook of Chronic Obstructive Pulmonary Disease

Handbook of Chronic Obstructive Pulmonary Disease

P John Rees, *MD, FRCP*
Sherman Education Centre,
Guy's Hospital, London, UK

Peter MA Calverley, *MB, FRCP, FRCPE*
University Hospital Aintree, Liverpool, UK

MARTIN DUNITZ

© 2002 Martin Dunitz Ltd, a member of the Taylor & Francis group

First published in the United Kingdom in 2002
by Martin Dunitz Ltd, The Livery House, 7–9 Pratt Street, London NW1 0AE
Tel: +44 (0) 20 7482 2202
Fax: +44 (0) 20 7267 0159
E-mail: info.dunitz@tandf.co.uk
Website: http://www.dunitz.co.uk

Although every effort has been made to ensure that all owners of copyright material have been
acknowledged in this publication, we would be glad to acknowledge in subsequent reprints or editions
any omissions brought to our attention.

A CIP record for this book is available from the British Library.

ISBN 185317-916-7

Distributed in the USA by
Fulfilment Center
Taylor & Francis
7625 Empire Drive
Florence, KY 41042, USA
Toll Free Tel: +1 800 634 7064
Email: cserve@routledge_ny.com

Distributed in Canada by
Taylor & Francis
74 Rolark Drive
Scarborough
Ontario M1R 4G2, Canada
Toll Free Tel: +1 877 226 2237
Email: tal_fran@istar.ca

Distributed in the rest of the world by
ITPS Limited
Cheriton House
North Way, Andover
Hampshire SP10 5BE, UK
Tel: +44 (0)1264 332424
Email: reception@itps.co.uk

Composition by Wearset, Boldon, Tyne and Wear
Printed and bound in Great Britain by Cromwell Press Ltd.

Contents

About the authors

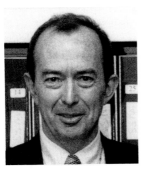

P John Rees

John Rees qualified from Cambridge and Guy's Hospital in 1973. He is a consultant physician and senior lecturer in general internal medicine and respiratory medicine. He has been involved in research related to asthma, COPD and sleep apnoea. In addition to original articles in these areas he is co-author of all four editions of the *ABC of Asthma*, co-edited the *ABC of Oxygen* series in the *British Medical Journal* and wrote *The Practical Management of Asthma* with Tim Clark. His other interests are in education as Site Dean for Guy's Hospital in the Guy's, King's and St Thomas' School of Medicine and Head of the GKT Department of Medical and Dental Education, London, UK.

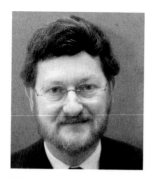

Peter MA Calverley

Peter Calverley is the Professor of Pulmonary and Rehabilitation Medicine at the University of Liverpool. He is a member of the Executive of the WHO/NHLBI Global Initiative in Obstructive Lung Disease and is an Associate Editor of the *European Respiratory Journal*. His research interests encompass a wide range of areas relevant to chronic obstructive pulmonary disease including its pathogenesis, diagnosis and effective treatment. He is past Chairman of the British Sleep Society and is currently investigating the cardiovascular impacts of sleep disorderd breathing.

Glossary

AAT	alpha-1 antitrypsin
CAO	chronic airways obstruction
CPAP	continuous positive airway pressure
CT	computerized tomographic
ECP	eosinophil cationic protein
EUROSCOP	the European Respiratory Society study of Chronic Obstructive Pulmonary disease
FER	forced expiratory ratio
FEV_1	forced expiratory volume in one second
FVC	forced vital capacity
IL	interleukin
IPPV	intermittent positive pressure ventilation
ISOLDE	the Inhaled Steroids in Obstructive Lung DiseasE study
KCO	carbon monoxide diffusion coefficient
LT	leukotriene
LTOT	long-term oxygen therapy
MMP	matrix-metallo-proteinase
MRI	magnetic resonance imaging
PEEPi	intrinsic positive end-expiratory pressure
PEF	peak expiratory flow
PM10s	small particulate matter

Foreword

This book comes at an opportune moment as chronic obstructive pulmonary disease (COPD) is rapidly rising up the medical and public health agendas. This is partly on account of the realization that it is an increasing burden on both the individual patient and society as a whole. As an example of this growing concern COPD is forecast to move up the ranks of mortality of disabling diseases as identified by the World Bank and it is now receiving attention from a number of sources including the World Health Organisation. It is also a disease whose turn has come to receive well-deserved attention having been overshadowed by asthma for the last two decades.

COPD is also coming under the scrutiny of government and public health departments because of associated rising costs and the need for coherence with anti-smoking programmes. It is also of growing interest to clinicians who realize the need to distinguish it from the other prevalent obstructive airway disease, asthma. This distinction is particularly important in elderly patients and in those who smoke tobacco with wheeze and dyspnoea. It is further noteworthy that the pharmaceutical industry has recognized these trends and is making major efforts to find new treatments as well as promoting existing ones.

For these reasons alone it is important to take stock and this book provides a useful addition to our growing body of knowledge about COPD. The Global Initiative in Obstructive Lung Disease (GOLD) has recently published its strategy document usefully summarizing the current science base of COPD with management recommendations. Professional societies such as the American Thoracic Society and European Respiratory Society are also considering how best to help their members keep up with growing knowledge and expertise on this rising burden of disease.

COPD is more than just a problem associated with smoking tobacco, although this does remain a central feature of its pathogenesis and avoidance. Many patients who present with a productive cough, breathlessness and wheezing have conditions other than COPD but taken as a whole this triad of symptoms presents major challenges to both clinicians and public health officers. This book provides an authoritative up-to-date account of COPD and should both add to the current knowledge as well as stimulate further plans to deal with this epidemic.

Professor Tim Clark, MD, BSc, FRCP, FCGI
Professor of Pulmonary Medicine
Imperial Colleage of Science,
Technology & Medicine
London, UK

Definitions

1

Introduction

Chronic obstructive pulmonary disease (COPD) is a major
cause of morbidity and mortality throughout the world and is
projected to be the third most common cause of death and the
fifth most important cause of chronic disability by the year
2020. The belated recognition of its social and economic
importance has led to a sudden increase in interest in the
diagnosis and management of this illness. A plethora of national
and international guidelines on diagnosis and management have
been published, which show a large measure of agreement
about the key diagnostic features. Representative of these is the
definition adopted by the British Thoracic Society:[1]

> 'Chronic obstructive pulmonary disease is a condition
> characterized by airflow obstruction ($FEV_1 < 80\%$
> predicted and $FEV_1/FVC < 70\%$), which is slowly
> progressive and does not change markedly spontaneously
> or in response to treatment.'

This type of definition is physiologically based and differs
significantly from earlier clinical and pathological ones that

led to the terms chronic bronchitis and emphysema.

Chronic bronchitis was defined epidemiologically as 'a cough productive of sputum for at least 3 months of 2 consecutive years'. This approach had the advantage of simplicity but did not take account of whether the sputum was purulent nor did it consider dyspnoea, the most important symptom prognostically and in terms of patient anxiety. The demonstration that prognosis was linked to the presence of airflow obstruction and not sputum production has led to the symptoms of chronic bronchitis being played down but they are important since they are the earliest features of the disease and a marker for early intervention.

Emphysema was defined pathologically as 'an enlargement of the terminal airspaces due to destruction of the alveolar walls without fibrosis'. This ignored the important effects of small airway damage and led to the unjustified assumption that the onset of dyspnoea was associated with this pathology. Recently, the development of high-resolution computerized tomographic (CT) scanning and the current vogue for lung volume-reduction surgery has stimulated a re-appraisal of the important role this process is playing at different stages of this illness.

The most recent definition of COPD is that offered by the World Health Organisation/National Heart Lung and Blood Institute GOLD initiative:[2]

'COPD is a disease state characterized by airflow limitation that is not fully reversible. The airflow limitation is usually both progressive and associated with an abnormal inflammatory response of the lungs to noxious particles and gases.'

This definition again emphasizes the fact that COPD arises because of the chronic exposure of the airways and alveoli to inhaled irritants, principally, but not exclusively, tobacco smoke.

Natural history

Information about the natural history of COPD is derived from a range of sources of variable reliability.[3,4] Mortality data usually comes from death certificates and reflects the prevailing patterns of terminology (Fig. 1.1). In contrast, morbidity data are derived from specific surveys which may or may not include measurements of pulmonary function. Despite these limitations, a reasonably clear pattern emerges.

Mortality

COPD is recognized to be of global importance, and is acknowledged by the WHO as the fourth commonest cause of death worldwide, with a mortality rate increase predicted for the next 20 years. In the UK, COPD accounts for 6–7% of deaths as a directly certified cause of death.[5,6] Total

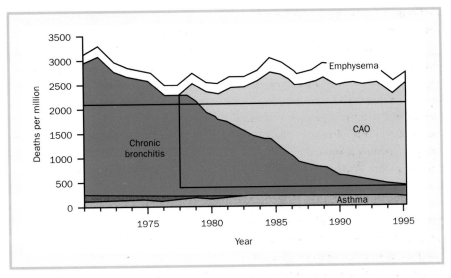

Figure 1.1
Total mortality from chronic obstructive pulmonary disease in England and Wales amongst older patients. Note that the overall number of deaths per million is relatively constant but the number attributed to different causes has varied with time. CAO (chronic airways obstruction) data derived from the Lung and Asthma Information Agency.

COPD mortality appears to be relatively constant in the UK over the last 20 years in the 65+ years age group (Fig. 1.1), although the overall number of COPD cases in all ages is falling. This reflects the cohort effect of the heavy smokers from the 1930s onward reaching their age of death. Nevertheless, the extent to which COPD plays an important secondary role in causing death is likely to be seriously underestimated, particularly when 'pneumonia' is the certified cause.

By the time patients are hospitalized with an exacerbation of COPD, they have a poor prognosis—especially if they have developed respiratory failure. In one unselected North American series of patients who were followed post-discharge from the ICU, one-third of patients had died within 12 months.[7]

Morbidity

Surveys in the USA indicate that 24% of Caucasian men and 20% of Caucasian women who smoke complain of chronic cough. The figures for obstructive pulmonary function tests are 15% and 10% respectively, and both are very much higher than the figures in non-smokers.[8]

The impact of COPD increases significantly with age. Thus the consultation rates with this diagnosis per annum in a range of general practices rise from 417 per 10 000 at ages 45–54 years to 886 at ages 65–74 years and reach 1032 in the 75–84-year-olds.

Early speculations that women were protected from COPD have proven ill-founded, indeed data from Scandinavia suggest that their mortality and morbidity is at least as great as that of men.[9,10] The present difference in symptoms and mortality reflects the later time at which cigarette smoking became common among women.

There is still debate about the role of chronic mucus hypersecretion in COPD. Although the initial finding that the rate of decline of lung function was independent of this is still generally held to be true, there is increasing evidence that hospitalization, especially for pneumonia, is commoner in those with a chronic productive cough.

Aetiology

This has been best studied in terms of factors that influence the rate of decline in lung function. Convincing evidence for the importance of tobacco smoking comes from the long-term follow-up in the UK by Professor Richard Doll and colleagues. The mortality from COPD was over 17 times greater in the smokers compared with non-smokers.[11,12] Fletcher and Peto,[13] in their classic study of UK postal workers, showed that the rate of decline of lung function (FEV_1) was greater in smokers (Fig. 1.3). Many other studies have subsequently found that the normal loss of FEV_1 of 15–30 ml per year increases to over 60 ml per year in current smokers and is still increased at approximately 40 ml per year in ex-smokers. Not all smokers develop this accelerated loss of lung function and conventional wisdom holds that only 15–20% of smokers are affected. This is misleading since it is very dependent on the age at which the populations are surveyed and more individuals will develop COPD as the population ages. Nevertheless, a range of factors other than smoking is likely to explain why some individuals develop disabling disease and others do not.

Progression

COPD is normally progressive, although it is unclear whether the rate of deterioration is constant in any individual. Blood gas tensions are usually preserved until the disease is advanced. Thus 40% of patients with an FEV_1 < 1.0 l will be hypoxaemic and this rises to 70% of those where the FEV_1 is 0.6 l. The onset of hypercapnia is often first noted during an exacerbation but when present persistently it carries a poor prognosis.[14] Weight loss is common as the illness becomes more severe and a low body mass index (< 19) is an independent risk for premature death.[15]

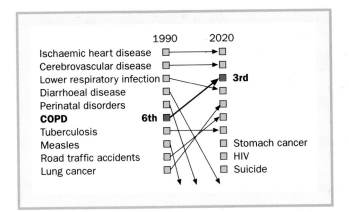

Figure 1.2
Future trends in chronic obstructive pulmonary disease mortality around the world. Data derived from Murray and Lopez.[6]

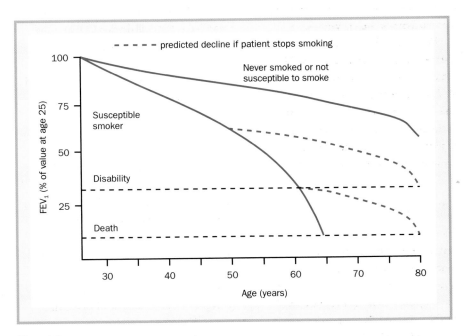

Figure 1.3
Age related decline in lung function. Note that these data begin from a standardized value at age 25 and do not take into account impaired lung growth due to smoking or other diseases. Modified with permission from Fletcher and Peto.[13]

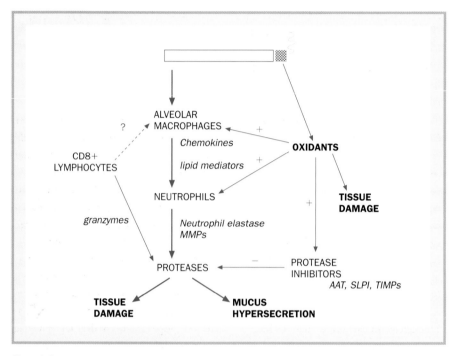

Figure 1.4
A possible pathophysiology scheme for lung damage in chronic obstructive pulmonary disease. Cigarettes cause recruitment of alveolar macrophages, which increase the proteolytic burden on the lungs causing tissue damage and excess mucus production. Direct damage by oxidants and indirect interference with these mechanisms is also important. + = augments the effects; − = inhibits the effects. Terms in italics are mediators produced by relevant cells or tissue damage.
MMP = matrix-metallo-proteinase; AAT = alpha-1 antitrypsin, SLPI = serum leucocyte proteinase inhibitor, TIMPS = tissue inhibitors of metalloproteinases.

Aetiological factors

As already noted, tobacco use, and cigarette smoking in particular, is the major identified cause of COPD in Western communities. Several other factors have also been identified either as important causes of COPD itself or closely related problems.

Genetic factors

The variability in the rate of decline in FEV_1 despite apparently similar tobacco exposures, together with the strong family history of obstructive lung disease in some families, suggest that polygenic mechanisms are likely to be operating. The best documented single gene mutation causing COPD is that of the α_1-antitrypsin gene, which was first described in Sweden over 40 years ago.[16] The substitution of a lysine for a glutamic acid residue produces a conformational change in the active site of the protein, which leads to polymerization in α_1-antitrypsin (AAT) as a β-pleated sheet within the hepatic mitochondria where it is synthesized. As a result, the protein cannot be transported into the circulation and the resultant low levels of circulating protein cannot protect against any excess of local protease activity, for instance from neutrophils in the lung. This autosomal recessive disorder is detected by the presence of low antitrypsin levels, typically in a young (< 50-year-old) patient. Only the homozygous ZZ form causes overt clinical problems, although recent data suggest that the MZ form is over-represented in patients undergoing surgery for severe emphysema. Smoking even a small amount can produce very severe COPD in these patients with extensive emphysema, which is predominantly basal.

Although several other gene defects, including the presence of specific polymorphisms for TNF_α and for aryl hydroxylase, which is involved in antioxidant defence, have been suggested as explaining the occurrence of COPD in the general population, these findings have been difficult to reproduce. Large genetic screening programmes in patients and their siblings are now beginning, in the hope of identifying new candidate genes.

Low birth weight and socioeconomic status

By the time most patients are diagnosed, the FEV_1 is reduced but this does not necessarily imply a very rapid rate of annual loss of lung function. It may be because they never reached their predicted pulmonary function before lung function began to decline and so they had a 'shorter distance to cover' before they became symptomatic — the so-called 'horse race' effect (see Fig. 1.3). Normally lung growth is maximal by the late teenage years, and lung function is relatively constant until the late 20s. Smoking teenagers do not achieve the peak values of their non-smoking contemporaries and begin to lose lung function as soon as growth ceases.

Any factor that reduces peak lung growth will predispose to COPD whether it is respiratory disease of prematurity, chronic untreated asthma or childhood malnutrition. In favour of this latter finding is the data reported by Barker and colleagues about the strong relationship of birth weight and lung function five to six decades later.[17] Whether specific malnutrition is the cause, however, is unclear since low birth weight is closely related to socioeconomic status. Whatever the explanation, enormous numbers of people worldwide are at great risk from COPD if they expose their already diminished pulmonary function to tobacco smoke.

Occupational factors

Chronic irreversible airflow limitation can develop after exposure to many agents that initially produce an asthmatic illness, agents such as toluene di-isocyanate (TDI), Canadian redwood cedar, and so on. The extent to which this type of exposure contributes to more usual forms of COPD is much less certain but there are increasing data to suggest that regular contact with organic dusts or chemicals increases the risk of airways obstruction, even when differences in tobacco exposure have been controlled for. Indoor pollution, particularly when cooking is performed in poorly ventilated homes, appears to be a major factor contributing to COPD in women in the developing world where tobacco use is still largely confined to men.

The most extensively documented occupational interaction is that with coal dust. Careful surveys over many years have found that exposure to coal dust in deep mine workers, especially those working when dust levels were very high 20 or more years ago, leads to an excessive loss of lung function above and beyond that expected with smoking. The decline of deep mining around the world with a switch away from fossil fuels is likely to make this once common problem of historical rather than practical importance in the future.

Bronchial hyper-responsiveness

For many years Dutch physicians have believed that COPD and asthma form part of a spectrum of illness, and that asthma in early life can progress to COPD later.[18] The pathological data argue against this type of overlap, which was determined by physiological testing. Long-term studies, however, such as the Lung Health Study in the USA, have reported a high incidence of non-specific bronchial hyper-reactivity to methacholine in people with mild COPD who smoke, especially in women.[19] This study does not establish whether this is a cause or consequence of smoking but follow-up studies should finally allow us to determine whether the presence of this type of 'asthmatic response' early in the illness predicts people who subsequently lose lung function more rapidly, as originally proposed by the Dutch.

Infection

The original British hypothesis that recurrent infection with purulent sputum caused progressive COPD was largely disproven by Fletcher and Peto.[12,13] CT scanning in COPD patients who complain of frequent episodes of cough and green sputum, however, has shown that a significant minority have evidence of tubular bronchiectasis. Childhood infection has not been found to be clearly predictive of future COPD once allowance is made for associated socioeconomic factors. Moreover, there is inconsistent evidence to indicate that some COPD patients have persistent lower respiratory tract colonization with common micro-organisms like *Haemophilus influenzae*. Whether this causes an accelerated loss of lung function is unknown. Observation of tissue from resected lungs has revealed the presence of adenoviral DNA incorporated in the genome as a latent form of viral infection. Tissue infected in this way shows an exaggerated degree of epithelial injury after contact with inflammatory stimuli like tobacco smoke. Further data about this intriguing process is awaited.

Pathogenesis

A range of theories have now been proposed to explain the processes by which COPD develops. The explanations are not mutually exclusive but lead to an emphasis on different potential targets for future therapies. Three major ideas now dominate thinking about mechanisms (schematically presented in Fig. 1.4).

Inflammation

The importance of persistent inflammation in COPD has been emphasized in the most recent WHO/GOLD definition (see earlier). In addition to the pathological data reviewed in Chapter 2 there are a wide range of observations from living patients to suggest that active inflammation is present. These factors include those listed in the following list.

- Elevated concentrations of TNF_α and IL-8, a neutrophil chemokine, in induced sputum from patients with stable COPD
- Increased numbers of all cell types and an increase in the percentage of macrophages and neutrophils in bronchoalveolar lavage specimens and induced sputum. There is no clear distinction between specimens from smokers with and without COPD in terms of the types of cell present but the numbers are always greater in smokers with established airflow limitation.
- Increased numbers of lymphocytes with normal or increased CD8 [T-suppressor] cells in endobronchial and peripheral lung biopsies. These cells are largely subepithelial and the number in the airway wall is correlated with the FEV_1, particularly when peripheral (small) airway tissue is studied. Some studies report slightly increased numbers of eosinophils but this is mostly related to exacerbations and is much less marked than in asthma.

The factors prolonging this persistent inflammation are only just being examined. A range of mediators including II-8, IL-6 and LTB4 have been found to be elevated in different COPD populations but no consistent story about which of the multiplicity of pathways is most important has yet been produced.

Protease-antiprotease imbalance

As noted in the context of genetic factors predisposing to COPD, deficiency of α_1-antitrypsin is associated with early-onset progressive emphysema. This observation made by Laurell and Ericson[16] over 30 years ago led to the development of the first biologically plausible explanation for the pattern of lung destruction seen in COPD. It was supported by animal experiments in which proteolytic enzymes where instilled intra-tracheally and, after a period of intense generalized inflammation, emphysematous lesions would develop. Studies using this model showed that this form of proteolytic insult could mimic the physiological abnormalities seen in severe COPD. Further studies showed that human neutrophil elastase was the principal source of proteolytic activity in established COPD, with specific effects on elastin, the principal structural protein in the alveoli. This led to the concept that, in COPD, the balance between the amount of elastase present in the alveoli and small airways was greater than the amount of anti-elastase, which usually protects the tissues. Cigarette smoke can oxidize the active site of the antitrypsin molecule (see later) and can cause chemotaxis of alveolar macrophages,

which themselves will recruit neutrophils and activate them within the airspace. Although α_1-antitrypsin deficiency explains relatively few cases of COPD, this concept of an increased elastolytic burden with a reduced defensive screen is an attractive one. Despite extensive study with a range of cellular and biochemical approaches, however, this remains a theory rather than an established fact. The opportunity of conducting a randomized controlled trial of replacement therapy (intravenous α_1-antitrypsin given every 2 weeks) has been lost at present since this is being given in an open study in the USA.

Recently another group of proteolytic enzymes, the matrix metallo-proteases, have attracted considerable attention. This group includes a number of collagenases as well as elastases and elegant studies in knock out mice showed that exposure to cigarette smoke only causes emphysema when these enzymes are present. Certainly they can activate neutrophil elastase and significant amounts of MMP's are released by alveolar macrophages An increased understanding of the interactions between these potent enzyme systems, the timing of their release and the role of oxidant processes should produce new therapeutic approaches to COPD within the next decade.

Oxidative stress

Cigarette smoke contains a high concentration of reactive oxygen species (ROS) (10^{17}

molecules/puff), and inflammatory cells such as activated macrophages and neutrophils also contribute. Evidence for increased oxidative stress in COPD is provided by the demonstration of increased concentrations of H_2O_2 in expired condensates and particularly during exacerbations, increased 8-isoprostane levels in urine and expired condensate.[20] The increased oxidative stress in COPD may have several deleterious effects; indeed, oxidation of anti-proteinases, such as α_1-antitrypsin and secretory leucoprotease inhibitor (SLPI) may reduce the antiproteinase shield, and may directly activate matrix metalloproteinases, resulting in increased proteolysis. H_2O_2 directly constricts airway smooth muscle in vitro, and hydroxyl radicals (OH^-) are potently inducers of plasma exudation in airways. Oxidants also activate the transcription factor nuclear factor-κB (NF-κB), which orchestrates the expression of multiple inflammatory genes, including IL-8 and TNF-α. Superoxide anions (O_2^-) combine rapidly with nitric oxide (NO) to form the potent radical peroxynitrite, which itself generates OH^-. Reactive oxygen species (ROS) also induce lipid peroxidation, resulting in the formation of additional mediators, such as isoprostanes and the volatile hydrocarbons pentane and ethane, as well as inducing DNA damage.

ROS are normally counteracted by both endogenous antioxidants (e.g. glutathione, uric acid, bilirubin) and exogenous antioxidants (e.g. vitamin C and vitamin E

from diet). There is, however, evidence for a reduction in antioxidant defences in patients with COPD who are more likely than control subjects to have a diet low in these antioxidant vitamins. Oxidative damage produced by cigarette smoke also causes stiffening of the neutrophil cell wall. This reduced deformability prevents these cells passing easily through the pulmonary capillary bed and encourages tissue migration. Recent animal studies have shown that the effects of cigarette smoke on lung structure and cellular activation can be blocked if recombinant superoxide dismutase is given at the same time as the smoke exposure. This is an important proof of principle but also highlights the ineffectiveness of most currently available antioxidants such as N-acetyl cysteine. This drug is widely prescribed in Europe as a mucolytic agent but is an excellent antioxidant in vitro. However, at the usually tolerated doses it is almost undetectable in the pulmonary tissues, which may explain its disappointing performance therapeutically.

Mucus hypersecretion

The two processes involved in mucus hypersecretion may have significantly different causes. The common complaint of increased sputum production is largely the result of increased secretion from hypertrophied mucus glands in the large airways. These show evidence of persisting inflammatory changes but the precise trigger for this is unclear. Ultrastructural studies of cilia in these airways show loss of ciliated epithelia and cilia that remain are short and thickened. This helps explain the impaired mucociliary clearance seen in COPD, which contributes to the accumulation of sputum. Cigarette smoke can have a direct ciliostatic effect, which may explain why sputum production is an early feature of this illness.

A second problem is the increased number and size of the goblet cells, which are distributed more peripherally. This does not necessarily produce more sputum but can contribute to peripheral airway plugging. Many of the enzymes thought to be involved in the genesis of COPD are potent secretagogues for mucus and cause goblet cell degranulation.

Comparison with asthma

As noted already, there are clear differences at a pathological, aetiological and clinical level between COPD and bronchial asthma. When the latter disease has progressed to the stage of significant airway re-modelling it can behave physiologically and clinically like COPD. Indeed, North American definitions of COPD have conceded this point by including such patients within this umbrella term. In most cases, the clinical presentations are relatively easy to distinguish. Key differences are:

- Clinical: most asthmatics present before the age of 40 years, have a childhood history of wheezing, are atopic, have intermittent symptoms with periods of well-being between times and have troublesome night-time and early morning cough and chest tightness. COPD normally causes symptoms of insidious onset in patients over 40 years, which are persistent and although varying from day to day are never entirely absent. The symptoms are present throughout the day and sleep disturbance is not a prominent feature. Breathlessness on exercise and then at rest gradually becomes the dominant complaint.
- Physiological: most asthmatics show substantial within- and between-day variability in lung function, whether measured as peak expiratory flow or FEV_1. If either value is reduced on testing administration of a short-acting inhaled bronchodilator will produce significant improvement, which normally substantially exceeds the minimal 15% and 200 ml change set arbitrarily as the limit of the bronchodilator response. Asthmatics commonly have a preserved or increased carbon monoxide transfer factor (DLCO) and exhibit exercise-induced bronchoconstriction. Non-specific bronchial reactivity to histamine and methacholine is normally increased. COPD patients have a persistently reduced

FEV_1, which is a better measure than peak expiratory flow (PEF) of the severity of airflow obstruction. They may show bronchodilator reversibility on repeated testing but this is usually modest with an absolute change seldom greater than 400 ml. Unlike asthma, bronchodilators do not restore the FEV_1 to within the predicted normal range. The DLCO is slightly to severely reduced in COPD, and exercise capacity is limited by the pre-existing airflow limitation, without further falls in FEV_1 post-exercise. The bronchial reactivity tests often show an apparent hyper-responsiveness but this arises for different reasons compared with asthma, a low baseline FEV_1 being a strong predictor of increased responsiveness.

- Pathological: these features are reviewed in Chapter 2 but studies of the inflammatory basis of COPD and asthma indicate substantial differences in the underlying cellular components with asthmatics showing a $CD4^+$ lymphocytic inflammation that is driven by allergic mechanisms, while COPD patients have a normal CD4:CD8 ratio or a relative predominance of $CD8^+$ lymphocytes in airway biopsies. Some of the relevant differences are summarized in Table 1.1.

Table 1.1
Differences between inflammatory response in asthma and COPD.

	ASTHMA	COPD
• Inflammatory cells	Mast cells Eosinophils $CD4^+$ cells (Th2) Macrophages +	Neutrophils $CD8^+$ cells (Tc) Macrophages +++
• Inflammatory mediators	LTD4, histamine IL-4, IL-5, IL-13 Eotaxin, RANTES Oxidative stress +	LTB4 TNF-α IL-8 Oxidative stress +++
• Inflammatory effects	All airways Airway responsiveness +++ Epithelial shedding Fibrosis + No parenchymal involvement Mucus secretion +	Peripheral airways Airway responsiveness Epithelial metaplasia Fibrosis ++ Parenchymal destruction Mucus secretion +++
• Corticosteroid response	+++	—

LT, leukotriene; IL, interleukin.

COPD is characterized by a neutrophilic inflammation, a large increase in macrophages and a preponderance of CD8$^+$ cells, whereas asthma is typified by an increase in active eosinophils, a preponderance of CD4$^+$ Th2 cells, a small increase in macrophages and mast cell activation. Whereas in COPD the predominant mediators are LTB4, IL-8 and TNF-α, in asthma LTD4, histamine, eotaxin, IL-4 and IL-5 are prominent. The inflammatory consequences between the two diseases are also different: in COPD there is squamous metaplasia of the epithelium; in asthma, the epithelium is fragile. The characteristic thickening of the basement membrane in asthma is not seen in COPD. There is parenchymal destruction in COPD that does not occur in asthma. Finally, the response to corticosteroids differs markedly between asthma and COPD, with an inhibitory effect of corticosteroids in asthmatic inflammation that is not seen in COPD.

Implications for the future

There is now a clear immunopathological difference between COPD and bronchial asthma which has not yet been translated into clinical terms. Using these discrete differences as a diagnostic tool is clearly cumbersome at present but it should finally allow resolution of the uncertainties about the effects of including asthmatic patients in large population series studying the natural history of COPD. Improvements in technology which allow the large scale and reasonably simple measurement of these important markers will undoubtedly have clinical impact but at present we are still reliant on a combination of clinical history taking, exposure to likely causative factors especially tobacco and pulmonary physiology in defining COPD.

Practical points

- COPD is a condition characterized by airflow obstruction (FEV$_1$ <80% predicted and FEV$_1$/FVC <70%), which is slowly progressive and does not change markedly, spontaneously, or in response to treatment (BTS definition of COPD);
- Chronic bronchitis is defined as cough productive of sputum for at least 3 months of 2 consecutive years;
- Emphysema is defined pathologically as enlargement of the air spaces due to destruction of the alveolar walls without fibrosis;
- COPD is the fourth commonest cause of death worldwide;
- COPD accounts for 6–7% of deaths in data from UK death certificates;
- Cigarette smoking plays the most important part in the aetiology, although other factors influence susceptibility and progression;

- Women are no less susceptible than men. Sex differences reflect differences in smoking rates in the past;
- Prevalence of COPD increases with age, around 15–20% of smokers develop COPD by the age of 60–70 years;
- The reasons for the increased susceptibility of some individuals are unknown, genetic factors are likely to be important;
- Homozygous deficiency of alpha-1-antitrypsin deficiency accounts for a small number of cases but illustrates an important pathophysiological mechanism;
- The inflammatory response in COPD shows clear differences from asthma.

References

1 British Thoracic Society. BTS Guidelines for the management of chronic obstructive pulmonary disease. The COPD Guidelines Group of the Standards of Care Committee of the BTS. *Thorax* 1997;**349**:1269–76.

2 www//goldcopd.com

3 Rijcken B, Britton J. Epidemiology of chronic obstructive pulmonary disease. *European Respiratory Monograph* 1998;7:41–73.

4 Strachan DP. Epidemiology: a British perspective. In Calverley P and Pride N (eds) *Chronic Obstructive Pulmonary Disease.* Chapman and Hall: London 1995, 47–67.

5 Murray CJ, Lopez AD. Mortality by cause for eight regions of the world: Global Burden of Disease Study. *Lancet* 1997;**349**:1269–76.

6 Murray CJ, Lopez AD. Alternative projections of mortality and disability by cause 1990–2020: Gobal Burden of Disease Study. *Lancet* 1997;**349**:1498–504.

7 Connors AFJ, Dawson NV, Thomas C, et al. Outcomes following acute exacerbation of severe chronic obstructive lung disease. The SUPPORT investigators (Study to Understand Prognoses and Preferences for Outcomes and Risks of Treatments). *Am J Respir Crit Care Med* 1996;**154**:959–67.

8 Center for Disease Control and Prevention 1998. Vital and Health Statistics: current estimates from the National Health Interview survey, 1995. DHHS publication no. (PHS) 96–1527.

9 Prescott E, Osler M, Andersen PK, et al. Mortality in women and men in relation to smoking. *International Journal of Epidemiology* 1998;1:27–32.

10 Prescott E, Bjerg AM, Andersen PK, et al. Gender difference in smoking effects on lung function and risk of hospitalization for COPD: results from a Danish longitudinal study. *European Respiratory Journal* 1997;4:822–7.

11 Doll R, Peto R, Wheatley K, et al. Mortality in relation to smoking: 40 years' observations on male British doctors. *BMJ* 1994;**6959**:901–11.

12 Peto R, Lopez AD, Boreham J, et al. Mortality from smoking worldwide. *B Med Bull* 1996;1:12–21.

13 Fletcher C, Peto R. The natural history of chronic airway obstruction. *BMJ* 1977; 6077:1645–8.

14 Costello R, Deegan P, Fitzpatrick M, et al. Reversible hypercapnia in chronic obstructive pulmonary disease: a distinct pattern of respiratory failure with a favourable prognosis. *Am J Med* 1997;**102**:239–44.

15 Landbo C, Prescott E, Lange P, et al.

Prognostic value of nutritional status in chronic obstructive pulmonary disease. *Am J Respir Crit Care Med* 1999;**160**:1856–61.

16 Laurell CB, Eriksson S. The electrophoretic alpha-1-globulin pattern of serum in alpha-1-anitrypsin deficiency. *Scand J Clin Lab Invest* 1963;**15**:132–40.

17 Shaheen SO, Barker DJP. Early lung growth and chronic airflow obstruction. *Thorax* 1994;**49**:533–6.

18 Orie NGN, Sluiter HJ, De Vries K. The host factor in bronchitis. In *Bronchitis, an international symposium.* University of Groningen, Royal Van Gorcum: Assen 1961, 43–9.

19 Kanner RE, Connett JE, Altose MD, et al. Gender difference in airway hyperresponsiveness in smokers with mild COPD. The Lung Health Study. *Am J Respir Crit Care Med* 1994;**4**:956–61.

20 MacNee W. Oxidants/antioxidants and COPD. *Chest* 2000;**117**(5 Suppl 1):303S–17S.

Pathology of COPD

2

Introduction

The pathological changes that occur in COPD reflect the effect of the inhaled insults, particularly tobacco smoke, which initiate the chronic inflammation that characterizes this condition. The distribution of this damage reflects the pattern of deposition of the inhaled particulates and the components within the tobacco which lead to tissue damage. The pathological changes arise from the interaction of the cells recruited by the inflammatory stimulus, and also the tissues that this stimulus affects. Thus although inflammation can be present in the small airways and alveoli, it produces fibrosis and airway narrowing in the former but tissue destruction in the latter. A further complicating factor is the interdependence between the tissues, which means that loss of elastic recoil as a result of emphysema can contribute to distortion and collapse in the small airways, which increases expiratory flow resistance. This makes it particularly difficult to derive simple relationships between measurements conducted in life such as the FEV_1 and the pathological abnormalities found, a problem which has not deterred many investigators from attempting this task!

As in many areas of medicine, our concepts about COPD have been greatly influenced by the tools available to gather information. The earliest descriptions of emphysema date back to the Scottish pathologist Matthew Baillie's description of Dr Johnson's lungs as being 'unable to deflate when removed from the thoracic cavity'. The accompanying lithograph suggests that emphysema was indeed the problem. These observations preceded the clinical studies of Laennec where the first good description of the clinical course of COPD was given. In contrast, descriptions of the pathological changes of mucus gland hypertrophy had to wait until the 1950s, although the term 'chronic bronchitis' had been in clinical use since the early 1800s. At this stage, the goal was to try and determine whether specific patterns of lung damage were associated with characteristic natural histories, an endeavour that left a large degree of confusion among pathologists and clinicians alike. During this time, from the 1960s to 1980s, autopsy data was complemented by surgical resection specimens, which allowed for the first time, good structure-function correlation studies to be undertaken. By the 1990s the technology of fibreoptic biopsy, bronchoalveolar lavage and, latterly, collection of induced sputum have been transferred successfully from bronchial asthma to COPD, and the emphasis has moved to understanding the immunopathological basis of the disease. This is reviewed in Chapter 1. Most recently, detailed quantitative studies have been performed on the nature of the inflammation in resection specimens from patients undergoing lung volume-reduction surgery. The results from these studies have challenged our previous ideas about 'end-stage COPD' being a 'burnt out' disease.

In this chapter, the patterns of damage as they occur within the lungs moving distally from the larynx will be reviewed, the pulmonary vascular and cardiac pathologies seen in advanced disease will briefly be addressed and some of the structure–function data that has influenced how we believe this illness evolves will be considered.

Central airways

The most consistent changes are squamous metaplasia of the epithelial surface without evidence of the sub-basement membrane thickening seen in asthma. Some cases have been reported where asthma-like markers, for example basement membrane thickness and concentration of eosinophil cationic protein (ECP), are increased in COPD patients who show an FEV_1 response to oral corticosteroids. This suggests that asthma and COPD can co-exist but more data are needed before this can be accepted as a robust concept. $CD45^+$ lymphocytes are seen in increased numbers with increased numbers of suppressor $CD8^+$ cells.[1] There are relatively few neutrophils present in airway biopsies, although some can be found trapped intraepithelially, possibly because neutrophils migrate directly to the airway lumen in response to chemotactic stimuli. Likewise, alveolar macrophage number are only modestly increased but large numbers of these cells are found in bronchoalveolar lavage specimens. Cigarette smokers without airflow obstruction show qualitatively similar but less pronounced changes. This pattern of inflammation extends from the trachea and main bronchi to the small airways (see later description).

Mucus glands are only present in the large airways but are increased in bulk. The ratio of the glands to the total diameter of the airway, the Reid index, is increased beyond the normal 0.26 to 0.59. The glandular structures are often infiltrated with inflammatory cells. Goblet cell numbers are increased and many show degranulation, changes that extend to the peripheral airways.[2]

Peripheral airways

The so-called small airways are defined as airways less than 2 mm in diameter without cartilage in their wall. They extend to the acinar structure of the lung and end at the terminal bronchiole. Marked inflammatory changes tend to be evident here before becoming obvious centrally. In advanced disease, there is marked distortion, oedema, fibrosis and smooth muscle hypertrophy of

these structures.[3] In this area, gas movement is no longer convective as in the central airways, rather it starts to become diffusive, increasing the contact time of the tissue and toxic gas. This situation is even more dramatic in the alveoli where some dilution with already resident gas occurs. Whether the concentration of toxic substances to which the small airways are exposed is greater than in the alveoli is unclear but in both areas it is greater than in the central airways, which may explain the distribution of tissue damage.

Alveoli

The characteristic lesion seen with exposure to cigarette smoke is centriacinar emphysema in which the central area of the respiratory acinus is destroyed around the respiratory bronchiole, with relative sparing of the peripheral acinar structures. Some patients, particularly those with α_1-antitrypsin (AAT) deficiency, develop panacinar emphysema with global loss of alveolar walls. Whether this is a truly different process or represents the evolution of earlier centriacinar damage is debated. The macroscopic lesions that occur when these lesions coalesce show a heterogeneous distribution, with the upper lobes dominantly affected in 'smokers emphysema' and the lower lobes usually predominating in AAT deficiency. Careful quantitative studies suggest that there is diffuse loss of alveolar surface area proceeding in parallel with the more obvious macroscopic damage, so that even the 'normal' lung adjacent to damaged areas may not be free from disease.[3] This helps explain the relatively brief (i.e. 12–24 month) benefits that follow lung volume-reduction surgery where macroscopically damaged areas are removed. It is likely that normal subjects show an increase in alveolar size as oxidative damage proceeds, and this effect of age will need to be allowed for when using CT scanning as a non-invasive method of studying the prevalence and progression of emphysema. This technique can now distinguish centriacinar from panacinar lesions, as well as identifying subpleural emphysema where pneumothorax is a possible complication. This is likely to allow us to make the first serial observations about the evolution of these lesions in subjects free of the inevitable selection bias of histopathological material.

There are now good data that emphysematous lesions are associated with increased numbers of inflammatory cells. The number of breaks in the alveolar walls and the reduction in attachments of the alveoli to the small airway walls correlate with the degree of inflammation. Studies from patients undergoing lung volume-reduction surgery have shown that, when allowance is made for the reduced amount of tissue present in these advanced cases, there is a remarkable increase in the amount of all types of inflammatory

cells, even eosinophils, as emphysematous lung injury progresses.

Pulmonary vascular and cardiac changes

The pulmonary capillary bed is destroyed in parallel with the extent of emphysema but, since there is an enormous amount of spare capacity in this system, there is no simple relationship between loss of capillaries and the severity of pulmonary hypertension at rest or during exercise. Detailed pathophysiological studies have shown that there is inflammation in the pulmonary arteries, even in early disease, that is very similar to that occurring in the adjacent airways and which is associated with local changes in ventilation–perfusion matching. In severe disease, there is thickening of arterial smooth muscle and reduplication of the elastic lamina with extensive pulmonary arterial wall re-modelling.[2,3]

In patients with persistent daytime arterial hypoxaemia secondary to COPD, the right ventricular mass is increased. This appears to be a compensation for the increased right ventricular work required in the face of a raised pulmonary artery pressure. The extent of the right ventricular hypertrophy is not, however, related to the pulmonary artery pressures measured in vivo, rather it is correlated with the usual arterial pressure of oxygen (PaO_2) experienced during the last year of life. This provides evidence that hypoxic vasoconstriction and secondary structural changes in the pulmonary circulation lead to right ventricular damage, which is described by the pathological term 'cor pulmonale'. Other changes associated with hypoxaemia are hypertrophy of the carotid bodies and an increase in the size of the glomerular tuft. Antemortem thrombus is often seen in the pulmonary arteries of those dying of advanced disease at autopsy, possibly secondary to local vessel wall irregularity and a chronic rise in plasma fibrinogen.[4]

Pathophysiological correlations

Several areas have been studied in detail:

- The relationship of pathology to clinical diagnosis;
- The relationship with pulmonary function;
- The relationship with gas exchange.

Relationship of pathology to clinical diagnosis

Many studies have examined the structural correlates of clinical diagnostic terms, generally with disappointing results. There is no relationship between the complaint of sputum production and the severity of the Reid index.[5] This is likely to reflect the lack of clinical precision in patients reporting sputum production, as well as the habit of some of swallowing rather than coughing up sputum. The relationship between emphysema and breathlessness is equally imprecise. Indeed the existence of discrete emphysematous and clinical subtypes, as postulated during the late 1960s, has been almost impossible to validate. Certainly, in some patients, either macroscopic emphysema or damage to the small airways appears to predominate but even here evidence of the other pathology can be found on careful examination. In most cases both processes are present, as would be expected given their common aetiology and the variable effects of dose of toxic cigarette smoke and individual susceptibility.

Relationship with pulmonary function

Studies measuring the distribution of airflow resistance in healthy subjects showed that only 20–25% of this lay in the small airways, a figure that rises to 70% in COPD patients. This means that significant amounts of lung function (as assessed by the FEV_1) are lost before the patient's problems are recognized clinically. There is an unresolved debate about whether this rise in peripheral resistance is principally due to damage in the small airways[6] or results from airway collapse secondary to reduced elastic recoil and airway distortion, as happens with emphysema. In truth both processes are likely to contribute.

There is good direct and indirect evidence that the severity of emphysema is well-related to the reduction in DLCO[7] (Fig. 2.1), although this relationship is lost when their FEV_1 falls below 1.0 and the DLCO becomes more difficult to measure. The factors leading to a rise in functional residual capacity are complex but there is increasing recognition that they are related to the severity of emphysema in many with advanced disease and that FRC can be reduced by removal of emphysematous lung.

Relationship with gas exchange

The original hope that patients who were 'blue and bloated' would have predominant 'bronchitis' while those who were 'pink and puffing' would have emphysema has proven false. There is no clear relationship between

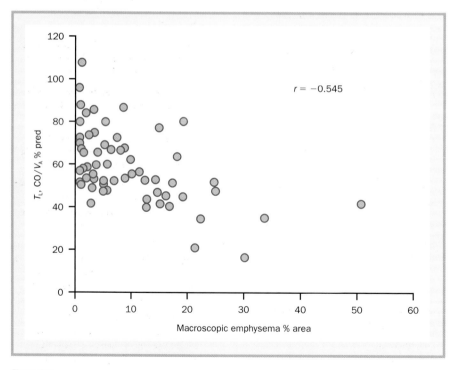

Figure 2.1
Relationship between carbon monoxide transfer factor (TLCO) per unit volume of lung and the amount of lung occupied by visible emphysema. Reproduced with permission from Gevenois et al.[7]

the extent of emphysema and the blood gas tensions. More elegant studies of gas exchange using the multiple inert gas elimination technique showed that patients with a high physiological dead space and high V/Q ratios were more likely to show extensive emphysema at autopsy. However, those with a large physiological shunt and a bi-modal V/Q pattern also included patients with extensive emphysema. Attempts to relate the presence of specific pathologies to desaturation during exercise have been equally unrewarding.

All of these studies indicate that the effect of structural damage in COPD is complex and can lead to the same physiological disruption by different but often overlapping means.

Practical points

- Pathological changes occur in central airways, peripheral airways and alveoli;
- In most cases changes are found at all three levels, although the relative proportions vary;
- Secondary changes occur in the pulmonary blood vessels and right heart;
- Enlargement of mucus glands and increased goblet cells are associated with increased sputum production;
- Narrowing and obliteration of peripheral airway contributes to the airflow obstruction;
- Cigarette smoke produces centriacinar emphysema, more marked in the upper lobes;
- Alpha-1-antitrypsin deficiency produces panacinar emphysema more marked in the lower lobes;
- Inflammatory cells are associated with the destructive lesions in COPD.

References

1 O'Shaughnessy TC, Ansari TW, Barnes NC, Jeffery PK. Inflammation in bronchial biopsies of subjects with chronic bronchitis: inverse relationship of CD8+ T lymphocytes with FEV_1. *Am J Respir Crit Care Med* 1997;**155**:852–7.

2 Lamb D. Pathology. In: Calverley P, Pride N (eds). *Chronic obstructive pulmonary disease.* Chapman and Hall: London 1995, 9–34.

3 Thurlbeck WM, Wright JL. *Chronic airflow obstruction* (2nd ed). BC Decker: London 1999.

4 Calverley PM, Howatson R, Flenley DC, Lamb D. Clinicopathological correlations in cor pulmonale. *Thorax* 1992;7:494–8.

5 Jamal K, Cooney TP, Fleetham JA, Thurlbeck WM. Chronic bronchitis. Correlation of morphologic findings to sputum production and flow rates. *Am Rev Respir Dis* 1984;**129**:719–22.

6 Hogg JC, Macklem PT, Thurlbeck WM. Site and nature of airways obstruction in chronic obstructive lung disease. *New Engl J Med* 1968;25:1355–60.

7 Gevenois PA, De Vuyst P, de Maertelaer V et al. Comparison of computed density and microscopic morphometry in pulmonary emphysema. *Am J Respir Crit Care Med* 1996;**154**:187–92.

Diagnosis and investigations

3

Diagnosis

The diagnosis of chronic obstructive pulmonary disease is based on a combination of clinical suspicion, the presence of appropriate symptoms and to lesser extent physical signs and the confirmation of chronic airflow limitation on objective testing. Patients are increasingly identified by the presence of abnormal spirometry undertaken for unrelated reasons e.g. as part of a general health examination or where COPD forms part of the differential diagnosis of another illness e.g. congestive cardiac failure.

Some patients are first seen by their family physicians or hospital specialist at an advanced stage in their illness and appear to have 'discounted' their symptoms for a long period of time before becoming acutely aware of them. This often follows an acute exacerbation but the mechanisms underlying this pattern of presentation are poorly understood. Much commoner is a presentation with respiratory symptoms which become progressively more intrusive. The intensity of the symptoms broadly parallels the decline in FEV_1 but the degree of an individual's health status impairment is not closely related to FEV_1 once COPD has become established. Thus for the same level of airflow obstruction some patients will complain of modest exertional breathlessness and others will be substantially disabled in their daily activities. How much this is associated with specific patterns of physiological abnormalities such as pulmonary hyperinflation and how much are recurrent exacerbations remains to be investigated. The pathophysiology of both symptoms and signs has been reported in details elsewhere.[1] The most important of these are discussed below.

Symptoms of COPD

Population studies such as the initial Lung Health Study have shown that many patients who smoke and have evidence of mild airflow obstruction (around 75% predicted) will nonetheless complain of cough or sputum production from time to time and sometimes as a constant physical finding. In the early phases of the disease, cough is constantly associated with the production of sputum, which may or may not be purulent. The volume of sputum is usually small and the cough is present throughout the day in contrast to the night-time predominance seen in asthmatics. These symptoms are worse in the presence of viral upper respiratory tract infection and the time to recovery from such events is longer than in patients without COPD. Patients acclimatise to these complaints and are often unaware that they are coughing. In patients with more established disease there is now evidence of a

reduced threshold to coughing as measured by inhaled capsaicin challenge. Patients who regularly produce dark green sputum are more likely to have associated bronchiectasis on CT scanning but in general the volume of sputum is low unless the bronchiectasis is very extensive. Patients producing clear sputum, yellow sputum or intermittently purulent sputum do not necessarily show the structural abnormalities.

Breathlessness is first noticed on vigorous exercise and the initial response is to avoid circumstances which lead to its production. As FEV_1 falls to 60% predicted patients commonly have difficulty maintaining the same walking speed as their contemporaries and may experience breathlessness during exacerbations. With worsening pulmonary function breathlessness comes to dominate the clinical presentation and is the most feared symptom by patients. The following features are usually present:

- Breathlessness is present throughout the day and may be associated with intermittent chest tightness, which must be distinguished from angina;
- Similar tasks will produce similar degrees of breathlessness on different days;
- The patient's appreciation of wheezing varies considerably and sudden attacks of wheezing are uncommon;
- Bronchodilator drugs appear to improve the rate of resolution of exertional

breathlessness but these effects are slower than in bronchial asthma.

Haemoptysis should never be attributed to COPD unless other causes have been excluded although it does undoubtedly occur from time to time. Weight loss is a feature of advanced disease but again other causes should be sought before accepting that COPD is the cause.

The striking feature about all the above symptoms is their persistence, particularly once the FEV_1 falls below 60% predicted. Although the patient may have 'good days' there are no prolonged periods when they are entirely free from breathlessness and capable of undertaking a level of activity equivalent to their fit contemporaries.

Signs of COPD

The physical signs in COPD are disappointingly non-specific although they are present if looked for carefully. In moderate to severe disease the patient may become cyanosed although this is notoriously difficult to establish in artificial light and a better marker for determining oxygenation is to measure arterial oxygen saturation or blood gas tensions when the FEV_1 falls below 35% predicted. Similarly weight loss may be evident and is particularly marked in the quadriceps muscle group. It is important to assess the legs of patients as this wasting may not be noticed if only the upper thorax is examined. Similarly a development of ankle oedema is an important marker of either co-existing cardiac disease or the onset of hypoxia-related pulmonary complications.

Many patients show features of over inflation of their lungs with horizontal ribs, splaying of the lower costal margins and a widened xiphisternal angle. In these circumstances, cardiac dullness is reduced on percussion and there may be occasional crackles and more commonly expiratory wheezes. However, the most consistent physical sign is a generalised reduction in the intensity of the breath sounds and this has been shown to be reproducible and to bear an approximate relationship with the forced expiratory time, itself a crude bedside indicator of reduced peak expiratory flow. Patients with more severe disease will be using their accessory muscles of respiration at rest and on careful inspection can be seen to be activating their abdominal muscles. This is commonly associated with paradoxical inward movement of the lower ribs (Hoover's sign) and may be accompanied by pursed lip breathing.

All of these clinical features can be present to varying degrees and tend to be more obvious when the patient is distressed during an acute exacerbation. Many patients with significant symptoms have none of the above physical signs and even if they are present there is always the need to conduct further investigation and so put the diagnosis on a firm basis.

Investigations

The extent of further investigation in COPD depends on the disease stage. Initial detection and assessment of severity depend on respiratory function, primarily spirometry. The place of the chest radiograph is largely to rule out other respiratory problems, particularly carcinoma of the bronchus in this high-risk group. In milder cases, no other investigations may be necessary. In more severe COPD, it may be appropriate to assess oxygen saturation or blood gases. Repeat investigations and other tests may well be appropriate in exacerbations, particularly if these are severe. Investigations include:

- Respiratory function tests;
- Radiology;
- Nuclear medicine;
- Blood gases, pulse oximetry;
- Electrocardiogram, echocardiography;
- Assessing quality of life;
- Assessing fitness for flying.

Airflow obstruction in COPD occurs as the result of several processes. There is increased mucus production in the larger airways and this is associated with persistent cough and sputum production but is not closely related to obstruction to airflow. The small airways in the lungs are also affected, showing narrowing, obstruction and obliteration. The total cross-sectional area of the airways (Fig. 3.1) increases markedly, going out through the divisions of the airways. In normal subjects only a small part of the total airways resistance resides in the small airways. Consequently damage to these small airways initially has little effect on airway resistance or symptoms. The early damage in susceptible smokers is not easily detected. As COPD develops and the damage to the smaller airways progresses airflow obstruction develops.

In addition to airways obstruction, the destruction of the lung tissue characteristic of emphysema leads to reduced elasticity of the

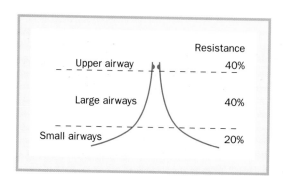

Figure 3.1
The cross sectional area of the bronchial tree from the larynx to the alveolar ducts. The resistance is split as shown. In the normal lung there is a great increase in cross sectional area at the small airway level which contribute only a small part to the total resistance. Considerable damage can occur at this level in a condition such as chronic obstructive pulmonary disease before there are any symptoms or detectable changes in conventional tests of lung function.

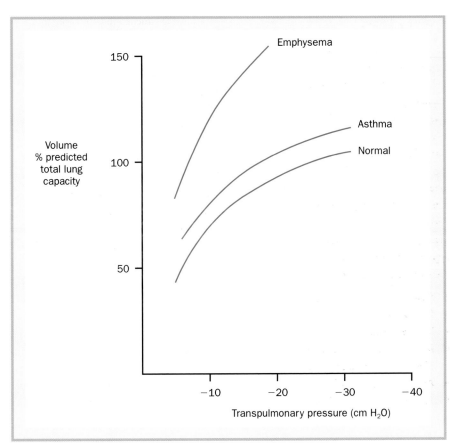

Figure 3.2
Static expiratory pressure volume curve in normal lung, asthma and emphysema. In emphysema the loss of elastic recoil in the lung means that larger volumes are achieved with a given transpulmonary pressure, shown by a change in the slope of the pressure-volume relationship and leading to a marked increase in total lung capacity. In asthma there may be an increase in TLC but this is much less marked and related to expiratory muscle activity, the slope of the pressure-volume relationship is not changed significantly.

lungs (Fig. 3.2) and loss of the supporting structure of the alveolar walls around the airways. Lung volumes are increased: total lung capacity; functional residual capacity; and, particularly, residual volume. In normal lungs, the volume at the end of a resting expiration is determined by the balance between the expanding force of the ribcage, which has a higher resting volume and the contracting elastic force from the lungs. In COPD, the elastic recoil of the lungs is reduced by the emphysematous change destroying the lung structure. In addition, airways may close off during expiration above this resting volume, resulting in the trapping of gas in the distal air spaces. The rate of emptying of the lungs is slowed and the next inspiration may start before all of the potential expiratory phase is completed. The increased

lung volume flattens the diaphragm, reducing its efficiency.

The loss of the alveolar attachments around the airways means that they are less supported (Fig. 3.3a,b) and more susceptible to the pressure around them. They may then collapse during expiration, particularly in a forced expiration and, in severe COPD, in a normal tidal breath. Patients may learn to reduce this airway collapse by pursed-lip breathing (Fig. 3.4), which maintains the pressure within the airways and resists collapse. Such collapse of the airways produces

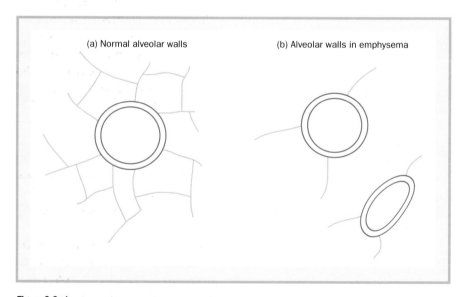

Figure 3.3a,b
(a) Normal alveolar walls and (b) alveolar walls in emphysema. Destruction of alveolar walls in emphysema increases lung compliance (reduced elastic recoil) leading to overinflation. The reduction in airways support leads to closure of the airways on expiration.

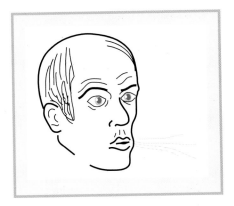

Figure 3.4
Expiration through pursed lips can help to prevent airway collapse. Many patients have learned to do this for themselves.

a pressure-dependent obstruction. This is seen during expiration but not inspiration, in contrast to the obstruction in a structurally narrow airway, which, although it may be affected to some extent by pressure changes across the wall, shows evidence of airflow limitation in inspiration and expiration. The collapse of the airways during a forced expiration explains why a forced vital capacity may produce a lower volume than a slow or relaxed vital capacity in emphysema.

Respiratory function tests

The most commonly performed respiratory function tests measure the degree of airflow obstruction during forced expiration. These

are used to grade the severity of disease in the published treatment guidelines for COPD.

Although measurements such as spirometry have become routine in COPD, the most important test for the patient is their ability to do everyday tasks and the associated limitations imposed on their life. Functional tests of walking or everyday tasks often correlate poorly with laboratory tests of respiratory function. Perhaps this is not so surprising since the forced expiratory manoeuvre is not part of normal breathing at rest or during exercise. However, the tests of expiratory airflow are simple to perform and remain important in the assessment of the patient with COPD. Whatever their relation to other measurements, they provide some indication of change with time and treatment. They form the basis of epidemiological studies of the effects of cigarette smoking and its cessation on COPD.

Spirometry

Spirometry is, therefore, more important than peak flow as a test of obstruction in COPD. Although equipment for spirometry has become more portable it is still relatively expensive and can rarely be given to patients to use at home, except for short periods or in research studies. This is less of a problem in COPD than asthma since short-term changes in obstruction are much smaller and the interest is more in the establishment of the

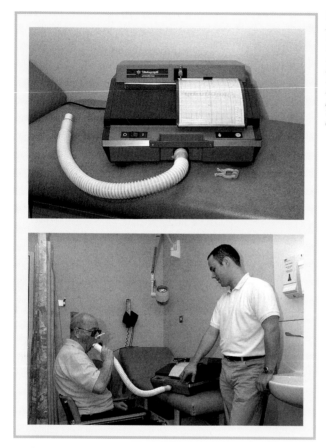

Figure 3.5
A dry-bellows spirometer such as the Vitallograph® is a robust machine suitable for measuring the relationship between volume in time in laboratories and surgery. Other machines based on a pneumotachograph or a turbine measure flow and convert it to volume.

degree of severity and in tracking longer-term changes. This makes a spirometer an important piece of equipment for all surgeries and clinics. Short-term changes may need to be assessed by a patient's response to bronchodilator or corticosteroid treatment.

A variety of equipment is available for measurement of spirometry. The robust standard is the dry bellows spirometer such as the Vitallograph (Fig. 3.5). Cheaper, more portable instruments based on a turbine vane or a pneumotachograph measure flow and integrate this to derive volume. Some of the simpler machines give a display of the

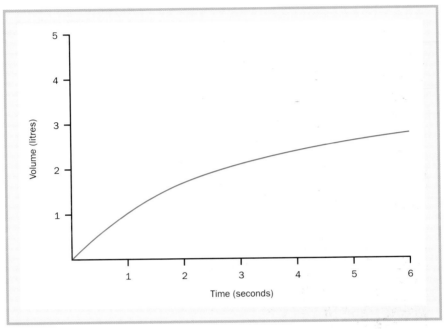

Figure 3.6
Volume–time trace in chronic obstructive pulmonary disease. The forced expiratory time is often greater than the 6 sec travel of a Vitallograph® carriage. As shown the trace is still rising at the end of 6 sec. Operators and patients need to be encouraged to continue to maximum expiration. In these circumstances a slow or relaxed vital capacity may be performed and produce higher values than the forced vital capacity since it reduces airway collapse produced by high intrathoracic pressure.

numerical values such as FEV_1 and FVC without a display of the volume-time curve or flow-volume curve. It is a great advantage to be able to see the shape of these traces to evaluate the adequacy of the expiration (Fig. 3.6) and to detect unusual abnormalities such as large airway obstruction where the expiratory flow rate is low and relatively fixed

(Fig. 3.7a,b). Some spirometers also allow the inspiratory limb to be visualized.

Spirometers should be calibrated regularly. This is usually performed with a gas syringe that is capable of pushing 3 l of air through the device at a representative flow rate. Frequency of calibration depends on the machine; to maintain accuracy it should

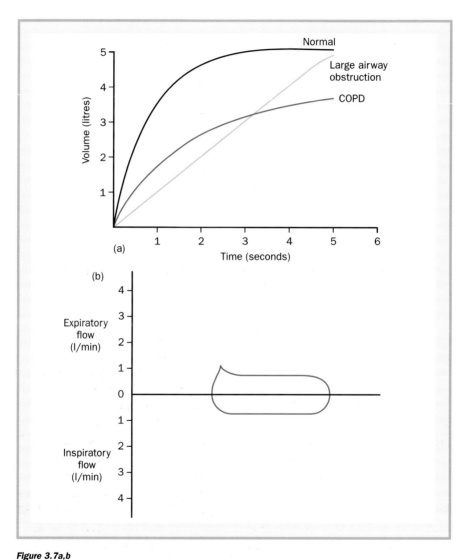

Figure 3.7a,b
In large airway obstruction such as a tracheal tumour there is a single fixed low flow rate throughout expiration and, consequently, a linear volume–time trace (a). This is more easily seen in a flow–volume trace (b) where the single low flow is more obvious. Comparison of the inspiratory and expiratory loop may indicate whether the level of the obstruction is inside or outside (e.g. larynx) the thoracic cage. In the example shown inspiratory and expiratory flow rates are the same indicating a rigid obstruction at either level.

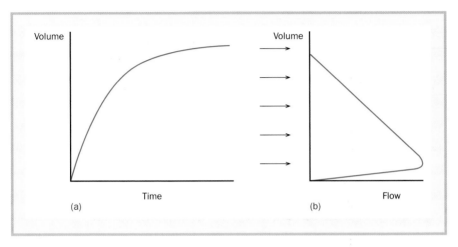

Figure 3.8a,b
(a) Volume–time and (b) flow–volume traces contain the same information. The flow-volume trace is conventionally displayed with volume on the horizontal axis.

usually be performed weekly for machines that measure volume and daily for flow-measuring devices.

The results can also be displayed as a plot of flow and volume (Fig. 3.8a,b). The normal curve has a brisk rise in flow to peak flow near total lung capacity then a steady decline down to residual volume. In contrast, the inspiratory limb is a smooth semicircle. With the development of disease in the smaller airways, the expiratory limb begins to dip at lower volumes. When a large degree of emphysema is present, there is a characteristic flow-volume loop with a sharp drop in flow after the initial peak, as the pressure in the thorax collapses the airways. This pressure-dependent

obstruction is limited to expiration and the shape of the loop on inspiration is near to normal, such that, at a given flow rate, there is much greater limitation of expiration than inspiration (Fig. 3.9a,b).

In COPD the length of the forced expiration is prolonged and can be a considerable effort for patients. The prolonged expiration with a positive intrathoracic pressure inhibiting venous return may cause dizziness or even syncope. A relaxed or slow vital capacity is obtained by a slow, steady expiration to residual volume. It is less of an effort for the patient. In normal subjects there is little or no difference between the relaxed and forced vital capacity. However,

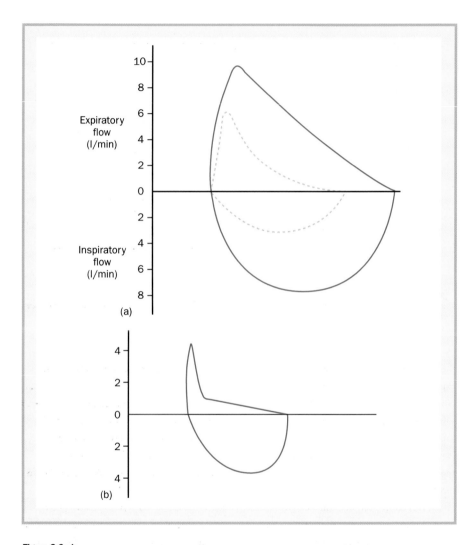

Figure 3.9a,b
Flow volume loops. (a) In chronic obstructive pulmonary disease (COPD) the first changes are a drop in flow rate at lower lung volumes resulting from changes in the small airways. Solid lines: normal; dotted lines: moderate COPD. (b) In emphysema much of the obstruction is dynamic, dependent on intrathoracic pressure. After an initial peak flow, the expiratory flow rate drops quickly to continue at a low rate while the inspiratory flow rate is relatively preserved.

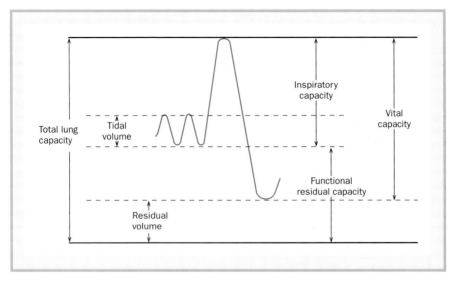

Figure 3.10
The divisions of lung volume. Measurements outside the vital capacity require instruments such as the body plethysmograph.

the collapse of the larger airways during forced expiration when there is substantial emphysema produces a forced vital capacity substantially less then the relaxed vital capacity. In practice, the relaxed vital capacity is not often used outside research studies in the UK. The FEV1 must be obtained on a forced manoeuvre but, to measure the FEV1 alone, this effort need not continue much beyond the first second. Other measurements such as inspiratory capacity avoid this pressure-dependent collapse and some studies have shown that they have a better relationship to functional measures of exercise but they are not used routinely (Figs 3.10, 3.11).

Accurate, reproducible spirometry requires careful attention to detail and considerable encouragement to the patient.[2] The ideal requires three reproducible volume-time traces. At least two of the FEV_1 values should be within 5% of each other. The curves should be smooth and free from irregular sections that suggest loss of sustained effort or coughing. During measurement of the FVC, the procedure must continue until all possible volume is exhaled. In patients with moderately severe COPD, this may take

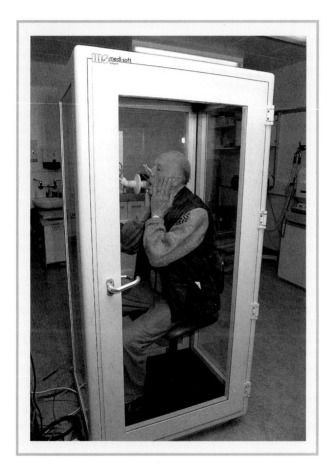

Figure 3.11
The body plethysmograph is used to measure lung volumes and airways resistance. The sealed system allows calculations of intrathoracic volume by the use of a derivation from Boyle's Law.

considerably more than the 6 seconds of movement allowed with a Vitallograph. Patients, nurses and doctors will need to be encouraged to continue the manoeuvre after the carriage movement has stopped to get the full expired volume. The results should be recorded as the best FEV_1 and FVC and compared with predicted normal values (which vary with age, sex, race and height).

A ratio of FEV_1 to FVC is termed the 'forced expiratory ratio' or FER. An FER of less than 70% indicates obstruction. If this ratio is over 70% and technically satisfactory, another diagnosis for breathlessness should be sought.

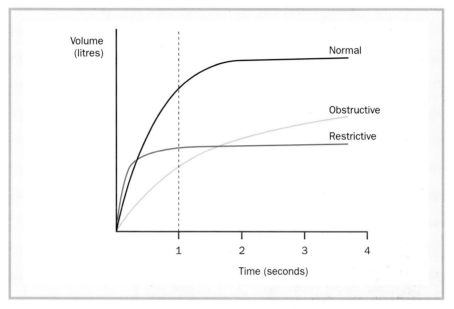

Figure 3.12
Spirometry (volume–time) traces in obstructive (e.g. chronic obstructive pulmonary disease) and restricitive (e.g. fibrosing alveolitis) conditions.

Normal, obstructive and restrictive spirometry traces are compared in Fig. 3.12.

The level of FEV_1 is the best predictor of future mortality and disability. In order to detect COPD patients with declining FEV_1 at a faster rate than normal (Fig. 1.3) accurate spirometry over some years is needed. Normal non-smokers have a drop in FEV_1 of 15–30 ml/year from the age of maximum lung function, which is around 25 years. To establish the rate of decline in an individual subject, recordings over at least 5 years are usually necessary (Fig. 3.13).

Peak flow

The main finding in COPD is obstruction to airflow. The most commonly used test for obstruction, familiar from the management of asthma, is the measurement of peak expiratory flow (PEF) by a peak flow meter (Fig. 3.14). Such measurements have the great advantage that they can be measured with a cheap portable machine. Many peak flow meters are cheap enough for patients to keep at home and they are available on prescription in the UK.

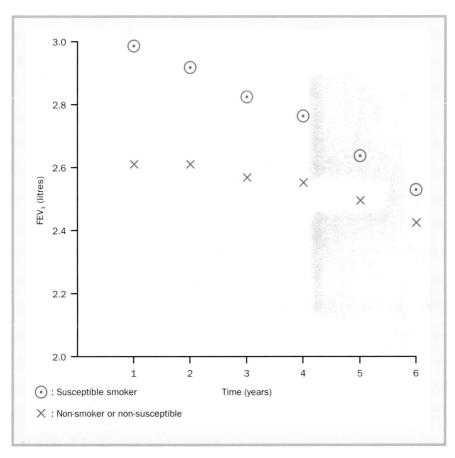

Figure 3.13
The 15% of smokers susceptible to the airway effects of cigarette smoking will have a decline of FEV_1 of around 50–70 ml per year. After the age of 25 non-smokers and non-susceptible smokers lose FEV_1 at 15–30 ml per year. The variabilty of the test means that measurements are needed over at least 5 years to determine the rate of decline in any individual subject.

Unfortunately peak expiratory flow is less useful as a measurement in COPD where the airflow obstruction is caused both by structural narrowing of the airways and by collapse of airways as a result of the positive intrathoracic pressure on forced expiration narrowing airways in floppy, emphysematous lungs (pressure-dependent obstruction). The

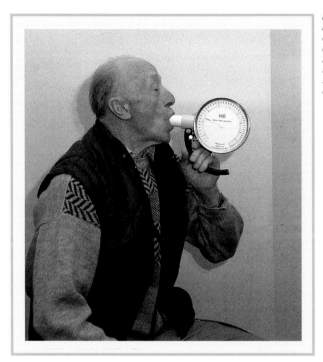

Figure 3.14
Peak flow is reduced in chronic obstructive pulomonary disease (COPD) but peak flow meters are more useful in asthma than in COPD where spirometry relates better to clinical severity.

peak flow rate may be relatively well preserved in such patients and the relationship to FEV$_1$ is poor.

Bronchodilator testing

Spirometry is often used to produce objective evidence of response to bronchodilators; however, there are several factors to consider. The first is the reproducibility of the test. In an individual patient a change of FEV$_1$ of 180 ml or FVC of 360 ml from baseline is outside the 95% confidence intervals of the test repeated over a short time period. In practice, this is taken as 200 ml in the FEV$_1$ and 350 ml in the FVC for statistically significant changes. A starting FEV$_1$ in severe COPD may be around 500 ml; this would mean an increase of 40% before the change can be confidently regarded as real. Responses can be presented in different ways (Fig. 3.15), for example percentage predicted etc. Spirometry is not the only measure of bronchodilator response. The subjective response and the ability to walk

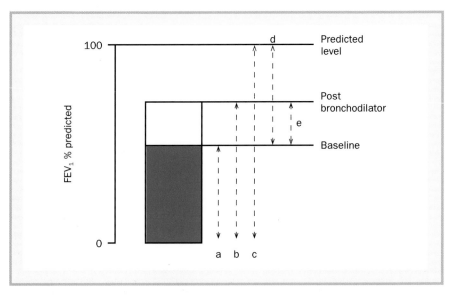

Figure 3.15
Effects of bronchodilator in chronic obstructive pulmonary disease can be expressed in various ways: absolute change: e = b − a; percentage change = 100 × e/a; percentage of possible change = 100 × e/d; change as percentage predicted = 100 × e/c.

further often do not relate closely to FEV_1 changes and all need to be taken in to account in deciding whether a response is likely to be clinically useful or not.

Bronchodilator responses are not always consistent. The failure to respond on one occasion may not fully predict the results of a subsequent challenge with the same drug. Nevertheless, the bronchodilator response can be useful in assessing the degree of reversibility. One of its most useful roles in the investigation of airflow obstruction is the diagnosis of asthma as suggested by a marked increase of perhaps 500 ml with bronchodilator therapy.

Responses to short-acting β_2 agonists such as salbutamol are taken at 15–30 minutes after administration of the inhaled drug while anticholinergic agents take 30–60 minutes to produce their maximum effect.

Transfer factor

The transfer factor test for carbon monoxide

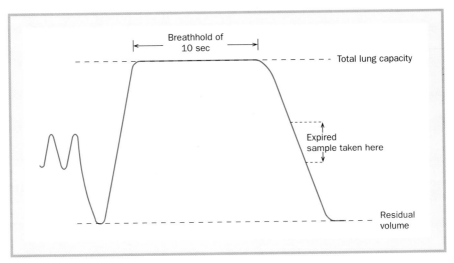

Figure 3.16
The single breath method for gas transfer involves inspiration of gas with a small known concentration of helium and carbon monoxide. On expiration after emptying the dead space a sample is collected for estimation of the expired helium (reduced by mixture with alveolar gas) and carbon monoxide (CO; reduced by mixture and by attachment of CO to haemoglobin in alveolar capillaries or free in alveoli).

(Fig. 3.16) measures the ability to move carbon monoxide from inhaled gas to haemoglobin in the alveolar capillaries. Carbon monoxide is used as a surrogate for oxygen. The gas mixture inhaled contains a small amount of carbon monoxide and a small amount of the inert gas helium. The helium concentration in the expired gas is lower than in inspired gas because of dilution with resident gas in the lungs. Carbon monoxide is reduced because of this dilution and transfer across the alveolar capillary membrane into the blood. The combination of the two allows an estimate of the amount of gas transfer into the blood. The result is expressed either as carbon monoxide transfer factor (TLCO) for the lungs or as transfer factor per unit lung volume accessed (diffusion coefficient or KCO). The KCO adjusts for the size of the lung accessed by the inspired gas, for example, a large pleural effusion will reduce lung volume and TLCO but not the KCO since gas transfer is normal within the lung accessed by the inspired gas. Asthma may reduce TLCO when severe but KCO tends to be high in asthma. Emphysema, with its

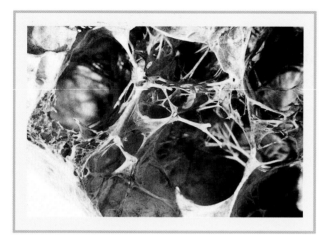

Figure 3.17
Loss of alveolar capillary membrane in chronic obstructive pulomonary disease (COPD) is one of the reasons for reduction in gas transfer in COPD. There is a weak correlation between the degree of emphysema and the reduction in gas transfer.

destruction of alveolar-capillary membrane, results in large air spaces (Fig. 3.17), decreased area for gas transfer and reduction of TLCO and KCO. In COPD, the reduction in KCO is a guide to the extent of emphysema. Other restrictive conditions such as fibrosing alveolitis reduce KCO but, within the obstructive lung conditions, reduced KCO is a marker for emphysema.

Lung volumes

The other respiratory test commonly performed in respiratory function laboratories is the measurement of lung volumes, residual volume and total lung capacity. These require more sophisticated equipment than spirometry since they have to measure the

volume of residual gas in the lungs that cannot be expired. The usual methods are to use an inert gas, usually helium, which distributes through this residual volume, and to measure its dilution or to use a sealed chamber, the body plethysmograph, where small changes in volume and pressure can be made during respiratory efforts. It is possible to obtain measurements of lung dimensions from posteroanterior and lateral chest radiographs and moderately accurate volumes can be calculated. A rough estimate of this is performed when overinflation is judged on the chest radiograph. However, it is not a suitable technique for repeated measurement and routine chest radiographs are not performed at completely maximal inspiration.

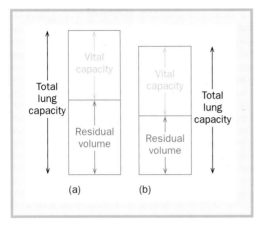

Figure 3.18
(a) before use of bronchodilators and (b) after. Bronchodilators may reduce overinflation without changing FEV_1 and FVC. This may explain relief of symptoms with bronchodilators without change in spirometry.

Body plethysmography

The helium dilution method and the body plethysmograph method can produce different values for lung volumes since the body plethysmograph measures all the gas within the thorax that is subject to the pleural pressure changes. The helium dilution only measures the volume accessible to inspired air. Poorly ventilated areas such as emphysematous bullae will be included in the plethysmograph volume but may not show on the helium dilution. This difference, the trapped gas, has been used as an estimate of extent of lung damage in COPD. After administration of bronchodilators the overinflation in COPD may be reduced. This can occur in the absence of significant changes in spirometry (Fig. 3.18). Such deflation can reduce symptoms of breathlessness or increase exercise tolerance and can explain subjective benefits found in the absence of any change in spirometry.

Other tests

Other tests such as flow-volume loops performed breathing a helium/oxygen mixture, closing volume of the airways or the frequency dependence of compliance have been used in research studies to look at the function of the smaller airways but have no established place in routine clinical practice. Measurements of respiratory system resistance and other variables related to small airways function can now be made using the technique of forced oscillation. This is simple and does not require patient co-operation but its role in the routine assessment of the COPD patient has still to be determined.

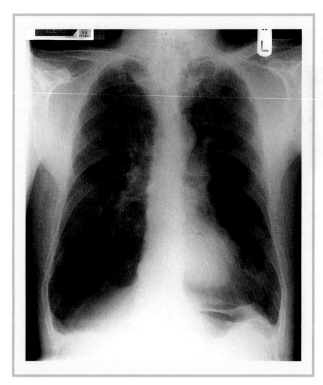

Figure 3.19
*The chest x-ray may show little
in chronic obstructive
pulmonary disease. However,
with considerable emphysema
the walls of bullae may be
visible as in this chest
radiograph. In this case they
are most marked at the bases.*

Radiology

Although the chest radiograph is regarded as a
standard investigation in COPD, it often
gives little valuable information about the
condition. Nevertheless, it is important as a
baseline measure for several reasons. Since
smoking is the main risk factor for COPD,
this group of patients is at high risk of
carcinoma of the lung. Occasionally the chest
radiograph may show extensive bullous

change (Fig. 3.19) not suspected from the
history or clinical examination. Overinflation
revealed on the chest radiograph is a more
common finding, judged from counting the
anterior ends of the ribs and the shape of the
diaphragmatic contours (Fig. 3.20).

In emphysema there may be a loss of
vascular markings in the lung fields; however,
unless emphysema is very extensive this is not
a reliable finding. At times of more severe
exacerbations, radiography may be useful to

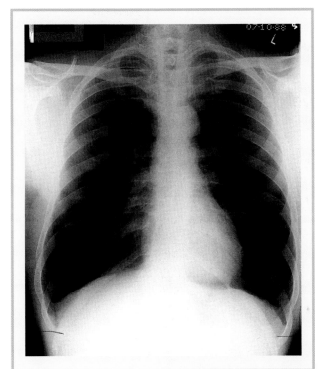

Figure 3.20
Hyperinflation is assessed on the plain chest radiograph by counting the anterior end of the ribs. In the mid-clavicular line on the right of the diaphragm should be at 6 to 6.5 ribs. Here the diaphragm is around the anterior end of the seventh rib.

identify areas of pneumonia (Fig. 3.21) or to look for a pneumothorax. Unless such problems are suspected there is little to be gained from repeating the chest radiograph routinely in COPD.

More sophisticated imaging such as computerized tomography (CT) has been used as a method of evaluating the extent of emphysema. This has been used quantitatively in research studies with accurate estimations of density of the lung tissue. More often, CT is used to evaluate the severity and distribution of emphysematous change. Discrete bullous change is easily seen on CT (Fig. 3.22) and is most important when lung resection is being considered, either for malignant disease or in the evaluation of patients for lung reduction surgery or removal of large bullae (see page 74).

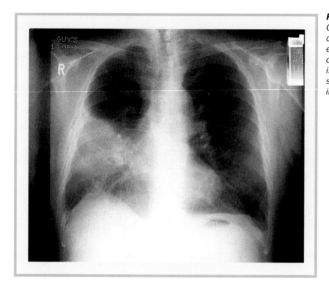

Figure 3.21
One of the reasons to take a chest radiograph during acute exacerbations of chronic obstructive pulmonary disease is to identify complications such as pneumothorax or, as in this case, pneumonia.

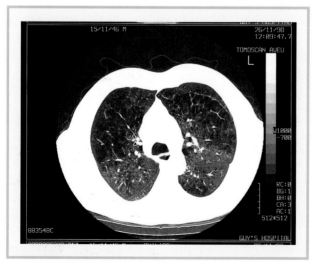

Figure 3.22
The extent and distribution of emphysema and the presence of bullae can be more easily assessed on computerized tomography.

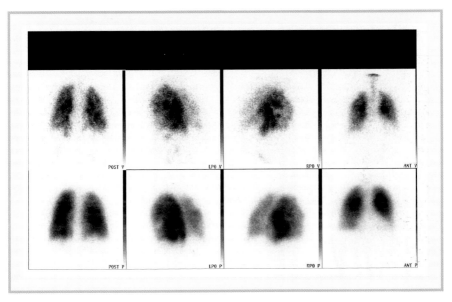

Figure 3.23
In chronic obstructive pulmonary disease ventilation perfusion scanning can be very difficult to interpret. There is patchy distribution of ventilation (upper row) and perfusion (lower row) in a matched fashion but mismatch representing pulmonary emboli will be difficult to detect.

Nuclear medicine

Lung scanning is not used routinely in the evaluation of COPD. When it is used in the search for suspected pulmonary embolism, the presence of COPD makes the interpretation of the scans much more difficult. COPD is associated with disruption of perfusion and ventilation in a partially matched fashion (Fig. 3.23). The typical pulmonary embolus pattern of reduced perfusion with maintained ventilation is then very difficult to identify

and the interpretation of the scan is usually guarded, necessitating some other diagnostic test such as spiral CT (Fig. 3.24) or pulmonary angiography if the suspicion of emboli is high.

Technetium^{99m} is used for perfusion and krypton^{81m} with a half-life of 13 seconds for ventilation. It is possible to use other isotopes such as xenon^{133} with a half-life of 5.2 days to quantify ventilation of areas of the lung and measure wash-in and wash-out characteristics but this is not used routinely in COPD.

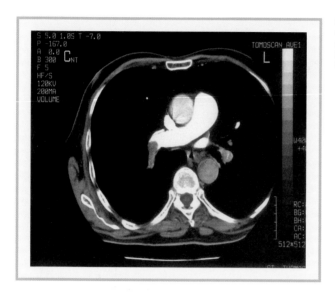

Figure 3.24
Spiral computerized tomography showing pulmonary embolus in the right pulmonary artery.

Microbiology

Most exacerbations of COPD probably have an infective origin and may be caused by bacteria or viruses. The commonest organisms are *Streptococcus pneumoniae, Haemophilus influenzae, Moraxella catarrhalis* (formerly *Branhamella catarrhalis*) and viruses. It is useful for microbiology laboratories to monitor the frequency and sensitivity of organisms cultured locally. In most exacerbations of COPD, management is not influenced by knowledge of the organism. In addition, the airways may be colonized chronically and isolation of an organism may not be evidence that it is responsible for an exacerbation.

Although antibiotics have been shown, in controlled trials, to confer some benefit, particularly in more severe exacerbations, the choice of antibiotic within a range of common, broad-spectrum drugs may not be important. Most microbiological information from sputum culture is only available after the patient begins to recover. It may help in episodes that respond poorly to initial treatment and in monitoring local resistance patterns. Therefore, when sputum is purulent and the exacerbation is moderately severe, it should be sent for culture. Sputum culture is also indicated when there is complicating underlying lung disease such as bronchiectasis or when pneumonia is suspected, when blood culture may also be indicated.

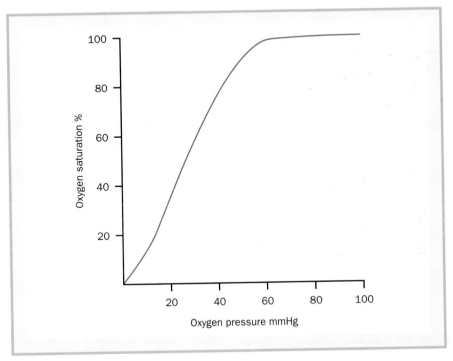

Figure 3.25
Oxyhaemoglobin dissociation curve. Saturation does not fall significantly until the partial pressure is well below normal.

Blood gases and oximetry

In the chronic stable situation blood gas examination is necessary to guide the provision of long-term oxygen treatment. In acute exacerbations, blood gas analysis helps to evaluate severity, prognosis and the need for oxygen treatment or respiratory support by invasive or non-invasive means. Blood gas analysis is still the only convenient way of

assessing $PaCO_2$ and should be considered in any patient with an FEV_1 below 1.21 or 40% of the predicted value or whose oxygen saturation is less than 92%.

Oximetry provides a measure of oxygen saturation and a portable oximeter is a very useful tool. The relationship between saturation and PaO_2 is given by the oxygen saturation curve (Fig. 3.25). Oximeters transmit light at set wavelengths through tissue in the finger or earlobe. Saturated and desaturated haemoglobin absorb the wavelengths differently and allow a calculation of the percentage of haemoglobin that is saturated. It is accurate in most routine clinical situations, although less reliable at saturations below 75%. When there is poor peripheral perfusion the signal may be inadequate or the reading inaccurate. In some circumstances, other pigments, such as nail varnish or carboxyhaemoglobin, produce inaccurate results.

Pulse oximetry (Fig. 3.26) provides a very useful measurement. It is important to remember, however, that it is only a measure of the oxygen level and does not provide a measurement of the level of carbon dioxide. In acute exacerbations, patients receiving supplemental oxygen may have marked carbon dioxide retention with an inappropriately reassuring oxygen saturation. In exacerbations requiring admission to hospital, baseline arterial blood gas analysis is usually necessary.

Assessment of blood gases are an essential part of the criteria for provision of long-term home oxygen. If the baseline oxygen saturation breathing air is above 92% then arterial PO_2 is not likely to meet the criteria. Oximetry therefore provides a useful screening test to see whether it is appropriate to go on to measure arterial blood gases.

Blood tests

A full blood count should be performed in the initial evaluation of moderately severe COPD and in more severe exacerbations. It may show polycythaemia in patients who are chronically hypoxaemic. If this is greater than expected from the daytime oxygen saturation there may be more profound nocturnal desaturation, perhaps related to associated obstructive sleep apnoea. The white count may be elevated in an acute exacerbation, especially if there is evidence of pneumonia. This may be more difficult to interpret, however, when corticosteroids have been administered since they may produce a neutrophilia in the absence of infection. Eosinophilia may suggest an asthmatic component to the airflow obstruction but eosinophils tend to disappear quickly with systemic steroid therapy.

In biochemical tests, liver function tests may be abnormal when there is pulmonary hypertension and cor pulmonale. Renal function may also deteriorate in cor pulmonale as a result of reduced renal perfusion, especially when diuretics or angiotensin-converting enzyme (ACE) inhibitors are used in the treatment.

The other test that should be considered is measurement of α_1-antitrypsin. The value of finding a low level is to intensify efforts to stop patients smoking, to consider replacement therapy and to look for other family members who may be affected. The measurement should be made by a quantitative test and should be performed when:

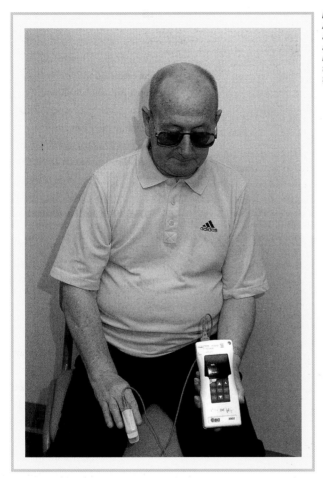

Figure 3.26
A number of oximeters are available. Some have the ability to record saturation over night, others are small enough to be carried during exercise tests.

- There is early-onset emphysema (below 50 years of age);
- COPD is diagnosed when smoking is minimal;
- The distribution of the emphysema is predominantly basal;

- There is a family history of α_1-antitrypsin deficiency or early-onset COPD;
- Cirrhosis is present with no other risk factors;
- Bronchiectasis is found with no other predisposition.

The measurement is best performed outside an acute exacerbation when the level may rise as part of an acute-phase response. If there is a low level of α_1-antitrypsin, the protease inhibitor genotype should be evaluated. Problems usually relate to the homozygous ZZ allele.

Electrocardiography and echocardiography

The electrocardiogram is not usually helpful in COPD. It may show evidence of P pulmonale (P wave >2.5 mm = 250 microvolts), a vertical or right-axis or right-ventricular hypertrophy (R wave in V1) but these add little to clinical findings.

The echocardiogram may be helpful in giving an estimation of pulmonary artery pressure. Other common echocardiographic findings in COPD are tricuspid regurgitation, right-ventricular wall thickening, increased right-ventricular volume and reversed movement of the interventricular septum. Nevertheless, overinflation of the lungs increases the retrosternal air space and creates difficulties in the performance of the echocardiogram in COPD. Consequently, it is often not possible to obtain adequate information.

Exercise tests

Estimation of exercise tolerance is part of a standard clinical history in patients with lung disease. Patients are asked to quantify their ability in terms of distance walked or stairs climbed. These need to be evaluated with care since many patients have poor judgement of distance. In outpatient practice breathlessness can be related to specific scales such as the 5-point Medical Research Council (MRC) dyspnoea scale. In studies of intensity of breathlessness during exercise, dyspnoea can be graded on a visual analogue scale or on the 10-point Borg scale between 0 = no breathlessness to 10 = maximal, the scale spaced so that a doubling of numerical score is related to a doubling of dyspnoea sensation.[3]

In research studies and most rehabilitation programmes, various types of formal walking tests are used. These are most commonly timed walks performed indoors on a flat circuit with standard encouragement where patients walk as far as possible in the time at their own pace. These were originally 12-minute walking tests but shorter walks of 6 minutes have been found to be satisfactory. They need to be performed carefully and there is a distinct learning effect increasing the distance achieved over the first few walks. A typical distance in a patient with an FEV_1 of 1 l would be 300–400 m. In very mild COPD, the test is not so discriminatory and in severe COPD motivation and expectations become more important in the test.

The 6-minute walking test requires a suitable, quiet, flat circuit without obstacles and it may be easier to provide facilities for a shuttle-walking test. In the shuttle test, an audible signal at increasing frequency defines the speed of walking around two markers at a set distance apart.

Formal cardiorespiratory exercise tests can measure gas exchange during exercise to find the maximal oxygen consumption. This can be useful in setting the initial level of exercise in rehabilitation programmes and in deciding on the limiting system in patients who have elements of cardiac and respiratory disease. They are performed on a bicycle or treadmill, measuring ventilation, heart rate, oxygen uptake and carbon dioxide production.

Health status and quality of life measurements

It has been recognized that objective tests of function and reversibility such as spirometry do not relate closely to subjective feelings of breathlessness or to ability to perform tasks such as walking. As in many other areas of medicine, increasing interest has centred on the effect of treatment on patients' quality of life, or health status. This should not be allowed to take over as the sole criterion since longer-term changes in the natural history of disease may be very important but not reflected in studies of quality of life even if these last a year or more.

In research studies, several questionnaires have been used to assess quality of life. Some of the most frequently used questionnaires are the St George's Respiratory Health Questionnaire (SGRQ)[4] and the Chronic Respiratory Disease Questionnaire.[5] The SGRQ is an extensive questionnaire designed to allow comparisons of health gain with therapy in COPD and asthma. There are three components covering symptoms, activity and impacts on daily life and well-being. The scale of the SGRQ is 0–100 with a change of 4 units estimated to equate to a clinically significant effect. The SGRQ is a long questionnaire, and abbreviated questionnaires such as the Respiratory Quality of Life Questionnaire (RQLQ) and the Airways Questionnaire 20 (AQ20) are quicker to use. The Chronic Respiratory Disease questionnaire was the first questionnaire specific for COPD. Four components cover emotion, mastery, fatigue and dyspnoea. It has been used to show change with treatment in short-term studies.

In addition, moderately severe COPD will produce abnormal findings on general questionnaires that are not disease-specific, such as the World Health Organization Quality of Life assessment instrument (WHOQOL-100), the Nottingham Health Profile, Sickness Impact Profile (SIP) and the Short Form (SF)-36 questionnaire.

Most of the questionnaires are used in epidemiological and other research studies. They have little use in everyday clinical management but the debate has emphasized the importance of matching the treatment and the evaluation of its effects to the needs and everyday experiences of the patient. A simple questionnaire that could be repeated in a clinic setting might become an established part of clinical assessment in the future.

Fitness for flying

Travel by land or sea presents few specific problems to patients with COPD. Those on oxygen may need to make arrangements for the availability of oxygen at their destination.

Air travel has become increasingly common over the last few years and patients frequently ask whether it is safe for them to travel and whether special arrangements need to be made about oxygen. Equipment such as nebulizers and nasal continuous positive airway pressure (CPAP) can be carried on aircraft but it is helpful to supply the patient with a letter verifying the need for medical use.

Some patients need supplemental oxygen during commercial flights. Most airlines pressurize their passenger aircraft to an equivalent altitude of 6000–8000 ft (1800–2500 m). This reduces the PO_2 of the ambient air to 15–18 kPa compared with 21 kPa at sea level. This worsens hypoxia in patients already hypoxic at sea level. In most patients this has no clinical significance.

Patients with resting hypoxaemia can run in to more severe problems with hypoxia if their starting PaO_2 is very low.[6] Relative

contraindications to flying are hypercapnia or gross hypoxia ($PaO_2 < 6.7$ kPa) equivalent to an oxygen saturation of around 85%. Various methods have been used; the most accurate method is to get patients to breathe a hypoxic gas mixture (15% oxygen, equivalent to an altitude of 7000–8000 ft) and to assess the blood gases. A simple screening test is to measure oxygen saturation breathing air at rest. If this is above 92% then breathing 15% oxygen or being at 7000 feet will not produce dangerous hypoxia and no special testing or flight arrangements are necessary. Regression equations based on spirometry and blood gases allow prediction of the effects of altitude but there is wide individual variation.

When the arterial oxygen falls to below 6.7 kPa (50 mmHg) breathing 15% oxygen, then oxygen should be available during a flight. This needs to be arranged beforehand with the airline, many of which make a charge for the provision of oxygen and can only do so if arrangements are made in advance. Patients on long-term oxygen therapy (LTOT) need their oxygen supplementation increased by 1–2 l/min during flights.

A current or recent pneumothorax is a contraindication to flying. The gas in such a non-communicating space will increase in volume at the lower pressure. Reasonable advice is to avoid flying for 2 months after a pneumothorax. Patients with emphysematous bullae that do not communicate well will be at increased risk of pneumothoraces but this alone is not usually a contraindication to flying.

Insurance policies should be checked carefully before flying since they may exclude treatment of a chronic condition such as COPD unless this is agreed beforehand.

Practical points

- Symptoms are persistent, show little variation and tend to worsen with time;
- Cough and sputum production are prominent early in the illness while breathlessness predominates later;
- The physical signs are non-specific until the disease is advanced with reduced breath sounds being the most reproducible finding;
- Spirometry is the main test of respiratory function used in COPD;
- Reproducible results require a careful approach to patient technique and machine maintenance;
- Lung volumes show increased residual volume and total lung capacity in COPD;
- Reversibility to a bronchodilator requires a change of around 200 ml in FEV_1 to be outside the variability of the measurement;
- Changes in spirometry relate poorly to changes in symptoms or walking distance in COPD;
- Some of the subjective changes may be related to reduction in overinflation without significant change in spirometry;

- One of the main functions of the chest X-ray in COPD is to exclude other significant disease;
- CT scanning can be used to evaluate the extent and distribution of emphysema;
- The disturbances in ventilation and perfusion in COPD produce difficulties in the diagnosis of pulmonary emboli by this technique;
- Sputum microbiology has little benefit for individual episodes but may help in defining the range and resistance patterns locally;
- Oxygen saturation by pulse oximetry is helpful but it is important to remember that it does not give information on carbon dioxide levels;
- Oxygen supplementation on flights should be considered when resting saturation breathing air is below 93%.

References

1 Calverley PMA, Georgopoulos D. Chronic obstructive pulmonary disease: symptoms and signs. *Eur Respir Monogr* 1998; **3**:6–24.

2 Quanjer PH. Standardised lung function testing: official statement of the European Respiratory Society. *Eur Respir J* 1993;(**Suppl 16**):5–40.

3 Borg G. Psychophysical basis of perceived exertion. *Med Sci Sports Exer* 1982;**14**: 377–81.

4 Jones PW, Quirk FH, Baveystock CM. The St George's Respiratory Questionnaire. *Respir Med* 1991;**85(Suppl B)**:25–31.

5   Guyatt GH, Berman LB, Townsend M, et al. A measure of quality of life for clinical trials in chronic lung disease. *Thorax* 1987;**42**:773–8.

6   Schwartz JS, Bencowitz HZ, Moser KM. Air travel hypoxemia with chronic obstructive pulmonary disease. *Ann Intern Med* 1984;**100**:473–7.

Prevention of COPD

4

Smoking cessation

The most important aetiological factor in COPD is smoking and the most important preventative measure stopping or, never starting, to smoke. In the UK, over 20% of adults continue to smoke regularly and rates in teenagers, especially girls, show little or no signs of decreasing (Fig. 4.1). In some developing countries, rates are increasing at a depressing rate (Fig. 4.2), storing up problems for the future with COPD and all the other smoking-related diseases.

The two important approaches concerning smoking and prevention of COPD are helping established smokers to stop and reducing the numbers who start smoking. Most smokers start in their teenage years. There have been great difficulties finding effective ways of preventing the onset of smoking in young people. The techniques need to be adapted to the age and social circumstances of the group being addressed. Peer, social and fashion influences have a great influence. Reduction in advertising, prevention of commercial targeting of young people and encouraging a responsible approach from role models may be the most helpful approaches.

Nevertheless, there have been successes in smoking

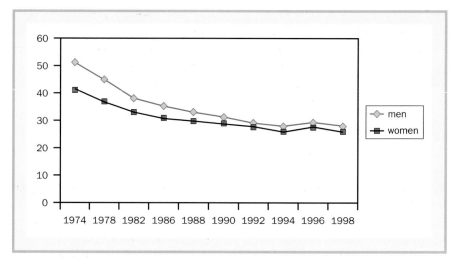

Figure 4.1
Prevalence of smoking in men and women in the UK from 1974 to 1998.

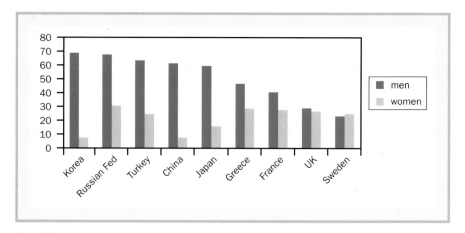

Figure 4.2
Estimated prevalence of smoking in men and women in various countries. There are marked differences between men and women in these countries.

cessation techniques, backed up by valid trials.[1] In established smokers, a wide variety of techniques have been employed. The simplest approach is to give basic advice on stopping smoking at each relevant health encounter, a surgery visit, appointment with practice nurse etc. Several studies have shown the success of this approach. Three minutes of advice is associated with 2% abstinence at 6 months compared with no advice. Although this may sound a low yield, the intervention is minimal and extremely cost-effective. Despite this, many smokers claim that they have never been given advice to stop, even during consultations related to their chest condition.

No techniques to help quitting are likely to be successful in smokers who are not motivated to stop, thus the first element may be to help to convince them of the benefits of stopping. Even with established COPD there are considerable advantages in stopping, ranging from a reduction in rate of decline of lung function, reduction in exacerbations and the ability to use treatment with home oxygen.

Simple advice that can be given in a brief consultation includes:

• Reinforcement of the benefits of quitting;
• Setting a date to stop;
• Telling people about the date;
• Seeking support of family and friends;
• Making a pact with doctor, nurse or family member to stop;

• Stopping completely rather than cutting down slowly;
• Linking stopping to other health changes, such as exercise, alcohol consumption;
• Keeping trying (most smokers do not stop at the first attempt);
• Considering nicotine replacement therapy.

Literature may be helpful to encourage smokers through this difficult period. Reinforcement by further contact and support will also be helpful but even this simple approach is helpful and is something to be considered at every consultation.

More intensive support is needed to produce higher cessation rates. Smokers' clinics with group support produce yields of abstinence at 6 months of around 8% compared with no intervention. A typical intervention would involve social support and training in coping skills with hourly sessions each week for 4–6 weeks and subsequent follow-up support.

Nicotine replacement therapy

The aim of nicotine replacement therapy (Fig. 4.3) is to replace the nicotine usually obtained from cigarettes, thus reducing the expected withdrawal symptoms. It results in an approximate doubling of cessation rates. In primary care this can increase cessation rates to around 10% and, in association with intensive intervention, cessation rates are

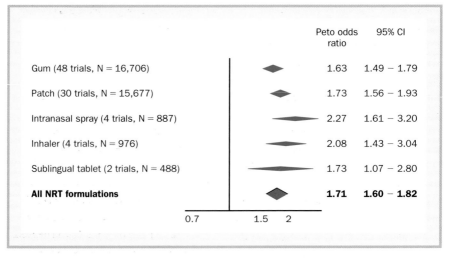

	Peto odds ratio	95% CI
Gum (48 trials, N = 16,706)	1.63	1.49 – 1.79
Patch (30 trials, N = 15,677)	1.73	1.56 – 1.93
Intranasal spray (4 trials, N = 887)	2.27	1.61 – 3.20
Inhaler (4 trials, N = 976)	2.08	1.43 – 3.04
Sublingual tablet (2 trials, N = 488)	1.73	1.07 – 2.80
All NRT formulations	**1.71**	**1.60 – 1.82**

Figure 4.3
Various forms of nicotine replacement therapy are available. Success rates are broadly similar for the different routes. The figure shows the odds ratios of 6 months abstinence for a meta analysis nicotine replacement strategies (reproduced with permission from Silagy et al[32]).

likely to be around 20%. Nicotine replacement is likely to be particularly beneficial if there are withdrawal symptoms on stopping. Withdrawal symptoms such as irritability, depression and urgency for a cigarette are reduced.

Several sources of nicotine replacement are available:

- Chewing gum: 2 mg and 4 mg doses are available in various flavours. Light smokers start with the 2 mg gum, while heavy smokers use the 4 mg gum. The gum should be chewed slowly;

- Patches: these are put on each morning and worn for 16–24 hours;
- Nasal spray: this produces a fast increase in nicotine levels. The spray may, however, irritate the nose but can be a useful adjunct to patches for heavily addicted smokers;
- Inhalator with a mouthpiece and nicotine cartridges: here nicotine is absorbed from the oral mucosa as with the gum.

Although the pattern of blood levels with nasal spray may mimic the cigarette smoke pattern, there is little evidence to favour one particular route. There may be benefits in a combination of therapies to maintain a background nicotine level with some rapid increases at times. Very few patients use nicotine replacement for the long term, even then they only maintain the nicotine intake, not the tar and carbon monoxide associated with continued smoking.

Trials of nicotine patch therapy suggest that 8 weeks treatment is as good as longer periods and that using the patch during 16 hours while awake is as good as 24 hours. Better results are obtained with the 4 mg gum in heavily dependent smokers. Theoretically a combination of patches and nasal spray might be most effective producing a steady background and the usual surges associated with smoking a cigarette. However, there is not convincing evidence of better results with combinations of nicotine replacement. It may produce better results in combination with bupropion.

In the United Kingdom at present nicotine replacement is available from pharmacies and, except for the nasal spray, without prescription. The costs are equivalent to the average costs of continued cigarette smoking. Nicotine replacement therapy became available on standard GP prescriptions in the UK in April 2001.

It is likely that nicotine replacement is safer than acquiring similar levels of nicotine by smoking in all situations. However, in the UK at present, nicotine replacement is not recommended in pregnancy and medical advice should be sought before it is used by patients known to have heart disease.

Bupropion

Bupropion (amfebutamone) is a drug that began life as an anxiolytic/antidepressant. Two large trials have shown that sustained release bupropion (300 mg/day) for 7–9 weeks, with supportive advice, improved cessation rates compared with placebo for up to the 12 months assessed in the studies.[4,5] Continuous abstinence rates for 12 months were 18% on bupropion and 6% on placebo. Symptoms of nicotine withdrawal were reported by the groups on bupropion but were significantly less than in the placebo arm of the study. A further advantage is that there was less weight gain in the bupropion than the placebo subjects. Insomnia and dry mouth were the only significant side-effects. Other side-effects of disturbance, rashes, headache and, rarely, seizures have been reported. There is some suggestion that the combination of bupropion with nicotine replacement therapy may be even more effective but further trials are needed. Bupropion, with appropriate advice, holds promise as a significant advance in smoking cessation management (Fig. 4.5). The dose is 150 mg/day for the first 3 days, and the quit date should be not immediate but 7–14 days after starting treatment. The second daily dose should not be in the evening to minimize problems with insomnia.

Caution is necessary in the elderly and those with liver or renal impairment. Bupropion should not be given to patients with a history or high risk of epilepsy. It should be avoided in pregnancy and breast feeding, in those with a history of eating or bipolar disorders, and in patients on ritonavir or monoamine oxidase inhibitors. Caution is needed for patients on antipsychotics, beta-blockers, Type Ic antiarrhythmics (propaferone, flecainide) or with drugs that lower seizure threshold such as theophylline.

Non-pharmacological methods of stopping smoking

Other non-pharmacological methods of treatment have been tried in helping smokers to stop. These include hypnosis, acupuncture, various relaxation therapies. In controlled trials, such interventions may produce short-term increases in cessation rates but are not generally associated with sustained increases in quit rates. They may help the motivation of smokers, particularly those who have tried unsuccessfully in the past, in which case there is little to lose other than the costs of the treatment and there is some suggestion that payment for the intervention may help quit rates, at least in the short term. However, the current recommendations that have the backing of established evidence concern simple advice, intensive support clinics, both backed up by nicotine replacement therapy

with the promise of further benefits from bupropion.

A monitor for carbon monoxide (Fig. 4.4) in the exhaled air will show whether smoking is continuing. Measures of continued smoking such as exhaled carbon monoxide or salivary cotinine are helpful in clinical trials of cessation methods. Use of such devices to confront continuing smokers may not be helpful but can be useful if used to show the effects of continued smoking and the return to normal values on quitting.

Weight gain after smoking cessation

Weight gain is a source of anxiety of many patients considering stopping smoking. Most of those who stop put on weight, partly because they eat more and partly because of better absorption. The average gain is about 7–14 lb (3–6 kg) but a few may gain much more. The health risks of the weight are much less than those of continued smoking but patients may find the weight unacceptable and young girls may smoke to restrict their weight. The possibility of weight gain should be acknowledged. An exercise regime in association with stopping smoking and being aware of the likelihood of increased calorie intake may help smokers limit the weight gain. Nicotine replacement therapy may delay most of the weight gain until the replacement stops and this may allow development of a regular exercise regime and the results with

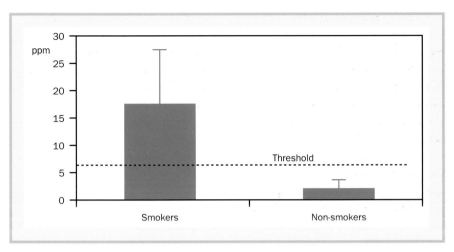

Figure 4.4
Carbon monoxide can be measured in exhaled air to give an estimate of carboxyhaemoglobin. This is a reasonable guide to recent smoking. Levels above 6 ppm strongly suggest current smoking (adapted from Middleton and Morice[3]).

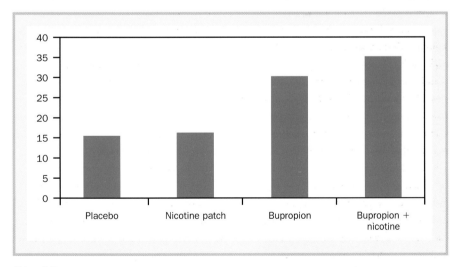

Figure 4.5
Abstinence rates at 12 months in a study comparing sustained relief bupropion with nicotine patch or a combination (adapted from Jorenby et al,[6]).

bupropion suggest that it may alleviate weight gain.

Environment

Outdoor pollution has been associated with exacerbations of asthma and COPD. Admissions to hospital are more common at times of higher levels of pollution. During the severe smogs of the 1940s and 1950s in cities such as London, high death rates from respiratory disease occurred among patients with COPD. Reduction in industrial and domestic generated pollution through regulation such as the Clean Air Act means that similar smogs are no longer seen. The reduction of levels of sulphur dioxide and smoke from coal burning has concentrated attention on other pollutants. Increased respiratory and cardiovascular admissions to hospital have been associated with nitrogen dioxide, ozone and small particulate matter (PM10s). Increased death rates have also been linked to higher levels of PM10s. It is difficult for individuals to do anything practical about outdoor pollution except to avoid exercising at periods of high pollution but the associations emphasize the importance of continued action on pollution, particularly in urban areas.

The indoor environment is also important in COPD. Indoor levels of NO_2 are often higher than outdoor and increase with poorly vented gas, paraffin and wood burning for cooking. These levels have not been studied so extensively as outdoor pollution. Attention should always be paid to the proper fitting and maintenance of cooking and heating appliances. This might be relevant to the development of COPD in some developing countries. It also applies to patients with established COPD who may be more limited in their ability to move out of their home.

α_1-Antitrypsin deficiency

In patients with α_1-antitrypsin deficiency it would seem logical to try to increase the levels of the deficient antiprotease. Attempts have been made to increase the levels by stimulating production. Danazol has some effect but the increases are insufficient to be of practical use. Since the abnormal enzyme is retained in hepatocytes, increased production might potentially increase the risk of significant liver damage. The recent findings on the crystal structure of α_1-antitrypsin show the structural changes that occur to retain it in the liver and raise the possibility of finding effective drug therapy.

The alternative approach is replacement. Human α_1-antitrypsin extracted from plasma is available in some countries but is expensive. It requires replacement through regular intravenous infusion. Recombinant α_1-antitrypsin has been produced but current molecules are less stable and have not been the subject of adequate trials of effectiveness or safety. Recombinant α_1-antitrypsin or another serum protease inhibitor might provide a cheaper replacement in the future.

There has not yet been an adequate controlled trial to demonstrate the benefit of α_1-antitrypsin replacement. It would be expected that this would be most useful as prevention before emphysema has developed. However, not all those with α_1-antitrypsin deficiency will develop emphysema. In some countries such as the USA, replacement therapy is now used quite widely where α_1-antitrypsin deficiency is detected.

The other consideration is whether replacement of α_1-antitrypsin to supplement the antiprotease/protease balance would benefit patients with cigarette smoking-induced emphysema with normal α_1-antitrypsin levels. At present there is no evidence that such replacement would be helpful.

Practical points

- Overall rates of smoking in the UK continue to decline slowly;
- Rates in young females show little evidence of decline;
- Simple, informed advice on quitting smoking from a health professional is associated with a small success rate but minimal cost;

- Weight gain often occurs on stopping smoking; diet and exercise should be addressed with advice on quitting;
- Nicotine replacement therapy more than doubles the success rates;
- Bupropion for 7 weeks with supportive counselling achieves 12 months continuous abstinence rates of 18%;
- Bupropion must be avoided in subjects with a history or high risk of seizures;
- The role of alpha-1-antitrypsin replacement remains uncertain.

References

1   Raw M, McNeill A, West R. Smoking cessation guidelines and their cost-effectiveness. *Thorax* 1998;**53**(Suppl 5):987–99.

2   Silagy C, Mant D, Fowler G, Lancaster T. Nicotine replacement therapy for smoking cessation. *Cochrane Database Syst Rev* 2000;2:CD000146.

3   Middleton ET, Morice AH. Breath carbon monoxide as an indication of smoking habit. *Chest* 2000;**117**:758–63

4   Hurt RD, Sachs DP, Glover ED et al. A comparison of sustained-release bupropion and placebo for smoking cessation. *N Eng J Med* 1997;**337**:1195–202.

5   Jorenby DE, Leischow SJ, Nides MA et al. A controlled trial of sustained-release bupropion, a nicotine patch, or both for smoking cessation. *N Engl J Med* 1999;**340**:685–91.

Overall approach to treatment

5

Introduction

The most important approach to COPD in the future is prevention. However, there are large numbers of patients who have already developed COPD, mainly from the effects of cigarette smoking. The current rates of smoking in most countries suggest that there will be a considerable need for treatment of established COPD for the foreseeable future.

Once COPD has developed, there has tended to be a negative approach to its treatment, on the basis that much of the problem is destruction of lung architecture that cannot be reversed. Although it is true that lung tissue damaged in the development of emphysema cannot at present be repaired, there is still much that can be done to prevent further damage, to prevent secondary complications of COPD and to relieve symptoms. Patients with severe COPD are very limited by their symptoms and feelings of frustration and even the development of depression are not uncommon. These may be reinforced by a negative attitude from health staff. Although repair of all the damage and return to normal function is not usually an option, every opportunity should be taken to approach management in a positive manner.

This chapter will give an overall approach to treatment dealing broadly with the desired aims of treatment. The way these have been gathered together into guidelines will be presented but the details of the individual treatments will be left to the chapters that follow.

Treatment strategy

Broadly, the aspects of treatment can be divided into:

- Prevention;
- Treatment of chronic stable COPD;
- Treatment of exacerbations.

Prevention has been dealt with in the previous chapter, and is concerned mainly with the avoidance and discontinuation of smoking. In the approach to the treatment of COPD, various attempts have been made to produce categories of severity. These are based on the degree of loss of FEV_1 compared with predicted values.[1] Although they generally relate to the severity of symptoms and the intensity of treatment, there is no strict rationale for the levels chosen, and some of the major international guidelines published over the last few years have chosen different levels. These have been used to guide the advice on categories of treatment within the guidelines.

The most frequently used sets of guidelines are those from the American Thoracic Society,[2] the British Thoracic Society[3] and the European Respiratory Society[4] (see Table 5.1). As with all guidelines new evidence becomes available before or soon after their publication and all three sets need to be reviewed in the light of more recent publications.

Table 5.1
Classifications of severity in the British, European and American guidelines for COPD: in each case the grading is as a percentage of predicted FEV_1 in the presence of a reduced FEV_1/FVC ratio.

	Percentage predicted FEV_1		
	British Thoracic Society	European Respiratory Society	American Thoracic Society
Mild (ATS Stage I)	60–79%	≥70%	≥50%
Moderate (ATS Stage II)	40–59%	50–69%	35–49%
Severe (ATS Stage III)	<40%	<50%	<35%

Treatment of chronic stable COPD

Within the management of chronic stable COPD there are various goals of treatment. These include:

- Prevention of further structural deterioration;
- Prevention of exacerbations;
- Prevention of secondary complications;
- Relief of symptoms.

In addition the role of surgery in COPD has come under new focus with the interest in lung reduction surgery. The modalities related to each of these are set out under the headings following. The details of the various modalities then appear in the chapters that follow.

Prevention of further structural deterioration

Several treatment modalities might appear under this heading. The most important is the avoidance of further exposure to the initiating causes of smoking and pollution.

Stopping smoking is the only intervention known to halt the damage of COPD in terms of the accelerated decline of FEV_1 and must be encouraged at every opportunity. Studies such as the Lung Health Study[1] have confirmed, in large groups that, on average, stopping smoking reduces the rate of decline of lung function to

that of a non-smoker (Fig. 5.1). This suggests that the process producing the lung damage of COPD has been stopped by removing the exposure. The slower annual decline of the non-smoker may still be important if a low level of lung function has already been reached producing symptoms from which even minor changes will be noticeable.

Limiting environmental exposure is important in some occupations with high levels of potentially damaging substances but is not known to be effective in other circumstances.

Knowledge of the underlying pathological damage, the mechanisms and inflammatory processes in COPD should lead to treatment that can affect the continuing damage. Proof would come from evidence that they reduced the rate of decline of lung function in COPD patients who continued to smoke, produced an improvement in lung function that was maintained on stopping the drug or, conceivably, prevented the annual lung function decline associated with ageing. Corticosteroids are the first obvious candidate in this area; however, although the large trials published recently have indicated beneficial effects from corticosteroids[5,6] they have not shown an effect on rate of decline of lung function. Attention is also being focused on other agents chosen from the growing knowledge about the pathophysiological processes involved in the development and progression of COPD.

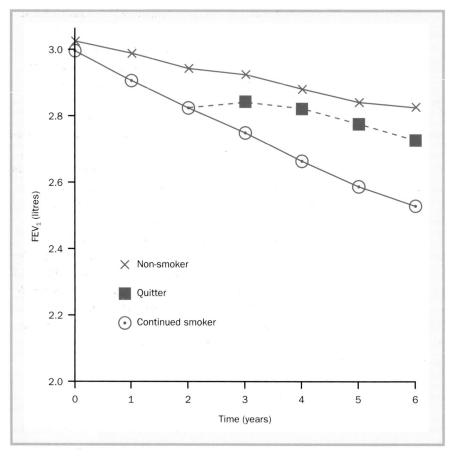

Figure 5.1
Stopping smoking arrests the faster decline of FEV_1 in susceptible smokers. There is little return of lung function but subsequent decline is at the slower speed of a non-smoker or non-susceptible smoker.[1]

Prevention of exacerbations

Most exacerbations of COPD are thought to be caused by infections, either viral or bacterial. Therefore, this seems the logical place to start with reducing exacerbations. Some of the problems in this area surround the definition of exacerbations, usually related to a combination of increased breathlessness, increased cough and change in sputum production. Most patients with moderate COPD appear to have between one and four exacerbations per year with a mean between one and two.

The two vaccinations that are most relevant are influenza vaccination and streptococcal immunization (see Chapter 7).

Influenza vaccination is the most effective way to prevent influenza and, in many countries including the UK and USA, is recommended for all patients over 65 years. Antiviral agents provide an alternative therapy as treatment of influenza.

Streptococcus pneumoniae is one of the three bacteria most commonly associated with exacerbations of COPD. The vaccine available has the potential to last 5 or 6 years and has been shown to be effective in younger people without underlying disease but at risk of streptococcal infection. Whether it works equally well in older people and in those with established COPD is more debatable. In the UK, vaccination is recommended for patients at risk such as those with COPD.

The other approach to infection would be treatment with antibiotics in a preventative manner. Antibiotics have been found to have an effect in the management of exacerbations (see Chapters 7 and 9). Antibiotics have also been tried as prophylaxis but have not found favour in the treatment of COPD. Exacerbations do not appear to be reduced in

frequency. They may be shortened in length but the same effect can be produced by the use of antibiotics at the first sign of an exacerbation. This approach is likely to be cheaper and less likely to lead to the development of resistance.

Short-acting bronchodilators do not seem to reduce exacerbations. There is more hope for agents acting on the underlying inflammation on the assumption that the infection associated with an exacerbation acts through an increase in the inflammation in the airway wall. Both antioxidants and corticosteroids have been claimed to result in a reduction in exacerbations of COPD. Results of two of the trials of inhaled corticosteroids (ISOLDE[6] and Lung Health 2[7]) indicate that inhaled steroids reduce the number of exacerbations (see Chapter 7). Long-acting bronchodilators may help reduce exacerbations.

Prevention of secondary complications

Secondary effects of COPD are related to the associated hypoxia and to the limitation in activity. The hypoxia associated with COPD leads to an increase in pulmonary artery pressure and to polycythaemia. The increased pulmonary artery pressure is one factor in the production of cor pulmonale with peripheral oedema and raised neck veins. In the right circumstances, oxygen therapy reduces this problem and improves the survival of COPD patients with significant hypoxia (see Chapter 10). Oxygen therapy also prevents secondary polycythaemia.

Diuretics and vasodilators are often used in these circumstances. They may provide some symptomatic relief but need to be used with care (see Chapter 10).

Loss of condition in non-respiratory muscles occurs in severe COPD when exercise tolerance is limited. Rehabilitation courses have been shown to be of benefit. Although it has not been tested in controlled trials it seems sensible to recommend maintained exercise from an earlier stage in COPD to prevent the deconditioning of muscles in the legs, trunk and arms. Attention to diet is also appropriate, avoiding obesity but maintaining adequate nutrition in severe COPD when weight loss may be a problem.

Relief of symptoms

The main symptoms of chronic COPD are breathlessness and cough with sputum production. The mainstay of symptomatic therapy has been with bronchodilators to relieve airflow obstruction and increase exercise tolerance. The effectiveness is less than in asthma but worthwhile improvements are certainly possible and should be pursued vigorously.

In addition, studies such as ISOLDE[6] have indicated that health status as measured by questionnaire can improve on regular inhaled corticosteroid treatment. Therefore these and possibly other long-term preventative therapy should also be considered to relieve symptoms.

In some circumstances, it may be appropriate to consider suppression of the cough with antitussives or relief of breathlessness by suppression of respiratory drive with opiates or anxiolytics.

Changing lung structure

Animal experiments are exploring the possibility of regrowth of lung tissue. At present, the only way to modify lung structure is surgically. Surgery for large bullae can be very successful. Lung transplantation is used in younger patients with very severe COPD. More recently, there has been attention in lung reduction surgery. The main aim is to remove very damaged lung to reduce lung volume, return a more normal and effective shape to the diaphragm and reduce breathlessness.

Lung volume reduction surgery has been evaluated in some small randomized trials.[8] Patients need to be very carefully selected. Results show improvements in lung function, walking distance and quality of life but the effects on mortality are uncertain.

The care of patients with COPD

Most cases of COPD are looked after in primary care for the majority of their illness.

Table 5.2
Clinical features of COPD according to grade and British, American and European treatment guidelines.

Grade (FEV$_1$ criteria differ in guidelines)	Clinical features	British Thoracic Society guidelines	ATS guidelines	ERS guidelines	Subsequent evidence
Mild	• Cough, with little or no breathlessness	• Inhaled bronchodilator as required	• β-agonist as required	• Inhaled bronchodilator as required • Influenza vaccination	
Moderate	• Breathlessness on on exertion	• Regular bronchodilators + oral steroid trial and consider inhaled steroids if positive • Consider long-acting inhaled bronchodilators, xanthines • Encourage exercise • Treat obesity or poor nutrition • Influenza vaccination • Identify and treat depression • Assess social circumstances • Assess for long-term oxygen therapy	• Regular anticholinergic+ β-agonist therapy as required • Consider xanthine or long-acting β-agonist • Consider mucokinetic agent • Consider oral steroid course and continue inhaled steroid if very effective • assess for oxygen therapy	• Increase bronchodilator treatment • Assess for oxygen therapy • Trial of oral or inhaled steroids, continue inhaled steroids if positive • Consider rehabilitation	More evidence available on long-acting, inhaled β-agonists • Effect of oral steroids may not necessarily predict those who will benefit from inhaled steroids
Severe	• Breathlessness on mild exertion or at rest • Cor pulmonale, polycythaemia	• Regular bronchodilators • Steroid trial • Assess for home nebulizer	• Increase bronchodilator therapy. • Rehabilitation		

Some specific tasks, such as more complicated lung function, blood gas assessment for long-term oxygen therapy or the management of severe exacerbations need to be performed as secondary care. As with most chronic diseases, however, regular, planned management by one or a few individuals provides the most effective pattern. This is often best performed by a nurse with training in respiratory medicine who can spend sufficient time discussing therapy, checking inhalation techniques and exploring areas such as diet, exercise and mood. This allows patients to build up confidence. Where there is a need for secondary care, a bridge can often be built by specialist nurses who work across between the hospital and the community in liaison with practice nurses in primary care.

When patients are admitted to hospital, the same specialist respiratory nurses can be involved in their care. Patients with acute exacerbations of COPD make up a significant proportion of general medical admissions, particularly in the winter months. In asthma it has been shown that the involvement of a respiratory physician, to look after the patient as an inpatient or during a consultation, improves the outlook and lengthens the time before readmission. It is likely that the same applies to COPD suggesting that respiratory physicians should have an involvement in the care of all patients with COPD admitted to hospital.

Practical points

- Prevention is the most important approach;
- Although much of the damage is irreversible most patients receive significant benefit from appropriate treatment;
- Severity is graded on the basis of FEV_1 but these boundaries are not absolute;
- Grading systems vary between different management guidelines;
- Stopping smoking is the only intervention known to alter the rate of lung function decline in smokers;
- Stopping smoking changes the rate of decline to that of a non-smoker;
- Most treatment is aimed at reduction in symptoms of breathlessness;
- A number of treatments, vaccination, inhaled steroids, long-acting bronchodilators show some promise in reducing exacerbations;
- Lung volume reduction surgery can produce significant temporary improvement in carefully selected patients;
- Management guidelines such as those produced by the ATS, BTS and ERS provide useful information on approaches to treatment (Table 5.2).

References

1   Anthonisen NR, Connett JE, Kiley JP, et al. Effects of smoking intervention and the use of an inhaled anticholinergic bronchodilator on the rate of decline of FEV_1: the Lung Health Study. *J Am Med Assoc* 1994;**272**:1497–505.

2   American Thoracic Society Statement. Standards for the diagnosis and care of patients with chronic obstructive pulmonary disease (COPD) *Am J Respir Crit Care Med* 1995;**152**:S77–S120.

3   British Thoracic Society. Guidelines for the management of chonic obstructive pulmonary disease. *Thorax* 1997; **52(Suppl 5)**:S1–S28.

4   Siafakas NM, Vermeire P, Pride NB, et al, on behalf of the Task Force. ERS Consensus Statement. Optimal assessment and management of chronic obstructive pulmonary disease (COPD). *Eur Respir J* 1995;**8**:1398–420.

5   Pauwels RA, Lofdahl C-G, Laitinen LA et al. Long-term treatment with inhaled budesonide in persons with mild chronic obstructive pulmonary disease who continue smoking. *N Eng J Med* 1999;**340**:1948–53.

6   Burge PS, Calverley PM, Jones PW et al. Randomised, double blind placebo controlled study of fluticasone propionate in patients with moderate to severe chronic obstructive pulmonary disease: the ISOLDE trial. *BMJ* 2000;**320**:1297–303.

7   Lung Health 2 Study. Effect of inhaled triamcinolone on the decline in pulmonary function in chronic obstructive pulmonary disease. *N Eng J Med* 2000;**343**:1902–9.

8   Geddas D, Davies M, Koyama H et al. Effect of lung-volume-reduction surgery in patients with severe emphysema. *N Eng J Med* 2000;**343**:239–45.

Bronchodilator treatment

6

Introduction

A major component of the treatment of COPD is control of symptoms. Although the degree of reversibility of airflow obstruction in COPD is limited, bronchodilators are a major component of this symptom control. Bronchodilators act mainly by relaxation of smooth muscle and the increase in airway calibre reduces resistance and can decrease the overinflation associated with COPD. Three groups of bronchodilators are available and, in addition to smooth muscle relaxation they have other potential effects, negative and some possibly positive, outside their bronchodilator action.

Assessment of bronchodilators

The common way to look at the effectiveness of a bronchodilator is by measurement of FEV_1 before and after administration of an inhaled short-acting agent. Short-acting β-agonists such as salbutamol or terbutaline are assessed 15–30 minutes after administration; the anticholinergic agent ipratropium bromide is assessed at 40–60 minutes. Three measurements of FEV_1 are made before and after. As explained in Chapter 3, the FEV_1 must change by 200 ml to be outside the variability of repeated measurements of the test (Fig. 6.1). The change is often expressed as a percentage change but 15% of a small baseline FEV_1 such as 0.6 l would be less than 100 ml and well within the error of the test, while 15% in a patient with mild COPD and an FEV_1 of 3.0 l would be 450 ml. Other criteria have therefore been proposed. The

American Thoracic Society criteria are an increase of 12% and at least 200 ml, European Respiratory Society criteria suggest 10% of the predicted FEV_1.

Although single tests of reversibility to short-acting agents are often performed, it has become evident that they are not always reproducible and often correlate poorly with symptomatic benefit. Since the drugs are being given largely for control of symptoms, the subjective benefit should play a major role

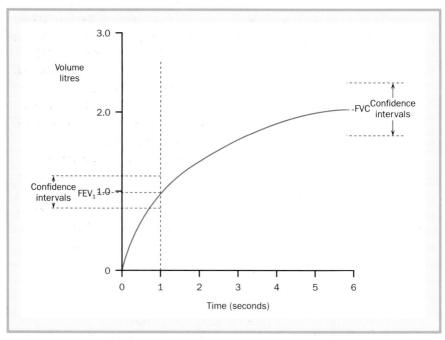

Figure 6.1
The variability of FEV_1 measurement requires a change of 200 ml to be sure it is outside the confidence intervals of the measurement. FEV change must be 350 ml to be outside normal variability.

in decisions on treatment. There are several reasons why the subjective effects and objective effects correlate poorly. One is that the small changes that are being measured in some patients and the tendency to want to dichotomize the effect into responders and non-responders. Another is the limitations of the FEV_1 measurement, which only measures one element of respiratory function and does not give information about other effects, such as reduction in overinflation. A number of studies have shown a disparity between the effects on walking distance and on spirometry.[1,2] A third component may be the other effects of bronchodilators; β-agonists may produce other noticeable sympathomimetic effects that influence a patient's judgement of effect. Despite these problems, assessment of bronchodilatation in single dose studies is useful since it gives an idea of the degree of bronchodilatation possible and the relation of changes to subjective effects. In some cases where reversibility is marked, it may raise the question of an underlying diagnosis of asthma rather than COPD and influence decisions about other treatments such as inhaled corticosteroids.

The single-dose studies should always be backed up by evaluation of the effects in longer studies looking particularly at effects on symptoms. For longer-acting agents, such as salmeterol or eformoterol, single-dose studies are inappropriate. Decisions should be based on the effectiveness of short-acting inhaled bronchodilators and confirmed by a trial of the agent for 2–4 weeks, which includes evaluation of subjective effects, including benefits on sleep, and, where possible, spirometry.

A reasonable regime for assessment of bronchodilator response is shown in Table 6.1.

This will help to determine what degree of reversibility exists at that time. It includes a reasonable dose of ipratropium bromide near the top of the dose–response curve in most patients. If there is a marked response to the β-agonist, the patient may fare better trying a β-agonist as a first-line bronchodilator rather than the ipratropium. This would then be followed by use of the chosen bronchodilator at home for 2–4 weeks before a further assessment of the effect on exercise tolerance and symptoms. In some patients with mild disease, the symptoms may be minor, such

Table 6.1
Scheme to assess bronchodilator response.

1. Take baseline measurements: take three FEV_1 measurements
2. Give 80 µg ipratropium bromide: at 45 minutes, take three FEV_1 measurements
3. Give 200 µg salbutamol: at 15 minutes, take three FEV_1 measurements

that they do not need a regular bronchodilator but just an inhaled agent to take when they feel breathless. Owing to the longer onset of action of ipratropium patients often feel the faster onset of β-agonists, salbutamol or terbutaline, more effective when used as required.

When regular bronchodilators are used it is often helpful to use an agent as background bronchodilatation, and give a short-acting agent for symptomatic relief in addition. The short-acting agent will usually be a β-agonist because of the speed of onset. There are three choices for the background dilatation:

1. A long-acting β-agonist (salmeterol or eformoterol) by inhalation or by mouth twice a day;
2. Ipratropium bromide or oxitropium bromide three or four times a day; or
3. A controlled-release theophylline orally twice a day. The introduction of longer-acting anticholinergic agents such as tiotropium[3] with a prolonged action allowing use once a day, will increase the options.

β-*Adrenoceptor agonists* (Fig. 6.2)

$β_2$-Receptors are found on airway smooth muscle from the terminal bronchioles up to the trachea. Their stimulation increases intracellular cyclic AMP, which activates protein kinase C, leading to the opening of potassium-activated calcium channels in the cell membrane. β-Agonists also act on mucous glands, pulmonary vascular smooth muscle, mucociliary clearance, some inflammatory cells and sensory nerves. Relaxation of vascular smooth muscle can potentially lead to a worsening of ventilation-perfusion matching in the lung and a reduction in PaO_2 as more blood flows to poorly ventilated alveoli. Occasionally, this can slightly worsen hypoxia in acute exacerbations but supplemental oxygen is usually being administered. Any effects of the other possible actions of β-agonists outside the airway smooth muscle are likely to be beneficial but the clinical significance is uncertain, the major benefit comes from relaxation of airway smooth muscle.

β-Agonists produce some degree of change in airway calibre in many patients with COPD at some time. In asthma, they are the most effective bronchodilator but, in COPD, most trials of single-dose or longer therapy show that anticholinergics produce a similar or greater effect. There are several considerations in such studies. Many studies have used conventional doses and the results have been variable. Some studies have given patients the dose for the maximal effect of one drug and observed the effect of adding the second agent. Some of these studies show no further effect, while some show that anticholinergics can produce a further benefit on top of the full β-agonist response. Interestingly, in acute exacerbations, when it

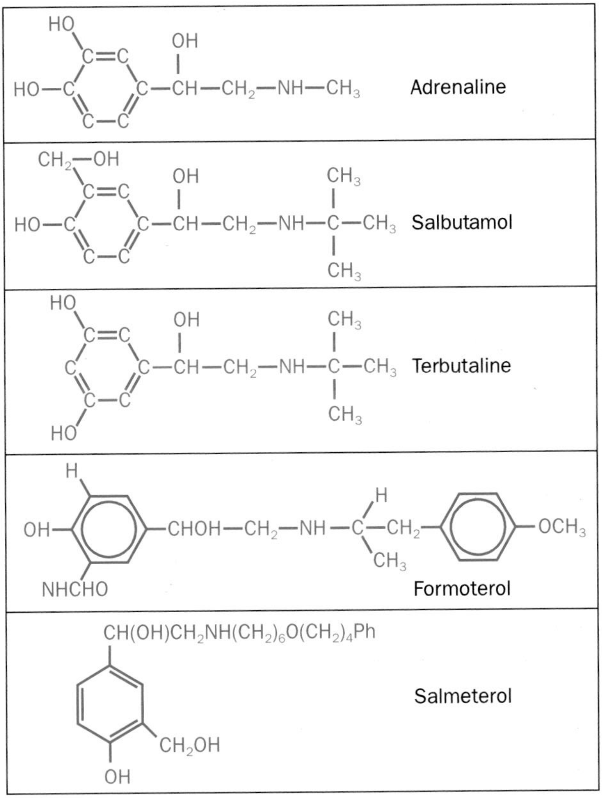

Figure 6.2
Structure of common short and long-acting ß agonists.

might be expected that a combination would be most useful, it seems that high doses of β-agonists and anticholinergics are equivalent, with no benefit from the combination.

In longer-term studies several other questions emerge:

• Are there any adverse effects?

- Are any initial bronchodilator effects sustained?
- Are there any effects on the rate of decline of lung function?
- Are other benefits or adverse effects affected by continued use?

Adverse effects

The most common adverse effects of β-agonists are tremor, tachycardia and hypokalaemia. In most patients, these are not a significant problem; however, some patients find the tremor or palpitations troublesome. Adverse effects often decrease and become tolerable with regular use but may prompt a change to an alternative bronchodilator. Hypokalaemia is a potential problem in patients on diuretics or with a tendency to arrhythmias, when care should be taken, especially with larger doses of β-agonists.

Sustaining initial bronchodilator effects

Several studies of asthma and COPD have suggested that there is some decrease in the bronchodilator effect with continued regular usage. The Combivent studies[4] over 90 days in COPD suggest a minor diminution in β-agonist bronchodilatation, which is not seen with the anticholinergic effect. However, such changes are very small, of dubious clinical significance and seem to reverse quickly on a short break from treatment.

Effects on the rate of decline of lung function

Some studies in asthma and COPD have suggested that regular bronchodilator use accelerated the rate of decline of lung function. However, the very large North American Lung Health Study[5] compared regular ipratropium bromide with placebo. There was no difference in the rate of decline of lung function, showing that there is no adverse effect on FEV_1 decline from regular anticholinergic use and raising considerable doubts about such an effect from β-agonists (Fig. 6.3).

Other benefits or adverse effects affected by continued use

Fortunately, although any decline in bronchodilatation with regular use is minimal, the adverse effects of β-agonists, such as tremor and tachycardia, are reduced by regular use. However, the same seems to be true for the protection against bronchoconstrictor challenge, which seems to decline with continuous use. Any relevance of this in COPD is uncertain.

Long acting inhaled β-agonists

In asthma long acting inhaled β-agonists have proved a useful addition to treatment. They have been shown to reduce symptoms and

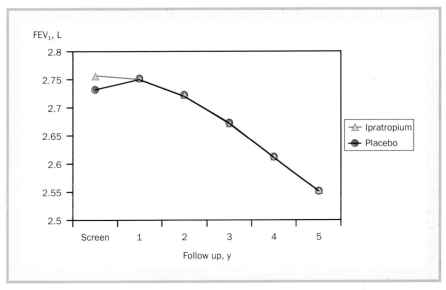

Figure 6.3
In the North American Lung Health Study regular use of ipratopium bromide had no effect on the rate of decline of FEV₁. There was a slight increase in the first year that was lost on discounting the bronchodilator at the end of the study (adapted from Anthonisen et al[6]).

improve quality of life (Fig. 6.4). In COPD, fewer trials are available; however, there is evidence of a beneficial effect with salmeterol and eformoterol with maintained bronchodilatation for 12 hours or more. The onset of action of eformoterol is faster than salmeterol but this makes little difference when the drug is being used as a regular twice a day bronchodilator for its sustained effect.

Salmeterol has been shown to produce a reduction in symptoms and improvement in lung function compared with placebo. One study has shown benefit from ipratropium and salmeterol used in combination.[6] Long-term studies of long-acting inhaled β-agonists, and combination studies with inhaled corticosteroids, similar to those in asthma, are awaited for COPD. In patients where there is a demonstrable benefit from short-acting β-agonists, and these are used regularly a long-acting β-agonist is a reasonable consideration. Its benefit should be assessed over 1 month or more of treatment that is based on symptoms and use of other

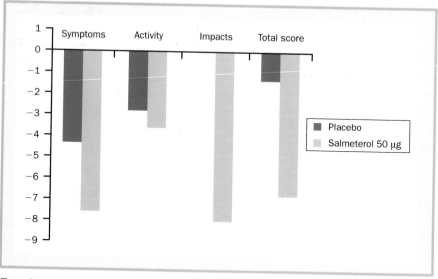

Figure 6.4
Salmeterol and formoterol have a bronchodilator action that lasts for 12 hours or more. Long-acting β agonists have been shown to have a significant effect on disease-specific quality of life measures such as the St George's Respiratory Questionnaire (SGRQ). The figure shows results for salmeterol 50 μg bd in a 16 week study. The threshold for a clinically significant difference in effect is 4 units. (Adapted from Jones and Bosh.[7])

treatment. The adverse effects are similar to those of short-acting β-agonists and the tolerance to the bronchoconstrictor protection without significant loss of bronchodilator effect also seems to occur with the long-acting agents.

Oral β-agonists

Although oral β-agonists are effective bronchodilators and tend to be cheaper than inhaled alternatives; they are not the preferred choice, since a larger amount of drug reaches the systemic circulation, and hence the body, from this oral therapy compared with inhaled products. The normal-release preparations of oral β-agonists therefore have no place in treatment; however, the newer long-acting preparations such as bambuterol can be useful, especially for nocturnal symptoms. They have the potential for more side-effects than inhaled drugs but they might be considered, particularly where cost or availability of inhaled drugs is a severe constraint.

Anticholinergic agents

For many years atropine was the anticholinergic agent used in airflow obstruction. It has been replaced by the quarternary ammonium compound, ipratropium bromide, which has fewer problems with potential extrapulmonary anticholinergic effects, such as drying of the mouth and exacerbation of glaucoma, which are theoretically possible but rarely of any practical importance. Cholinergic receptors are found on the smooth muscle of the larger airways, but much less so in smaller airways, making them less widely distributed than β-agonist receptors. Five types of human muscarinic receptors have been identified and those in the airway are of three main types (Fig. 6.5):

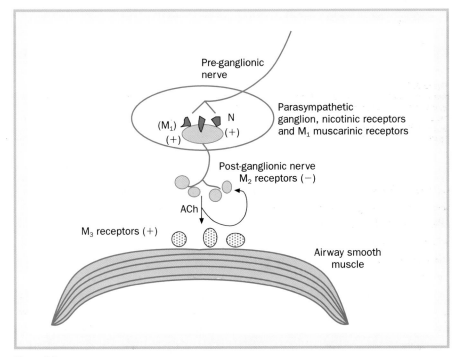

Figure 6.5
Muscarinic receptor subtypes in the human airway. Current anticholinergic drugs are not specific. Drug specific for M_1 receptors might avoid the negative feedback of M_2 receptors on the postganglionic nerve.

- M_1 in the parasympathetic ganglion, facilitate cholinergic neurotransmission and enhance cholinergic bronchoconstriction;
- M_2 on cholinergic nerve endings inhibit release of acetylcholine acting negatively on receptors in the postganglionic nerve. Blockade increases acetylcholine release;
- M_3 on airways smooth muscle and glands produce bronchoconstriction and mucus secretion.

Currently available drugs such as atropine and ipratropium bromide are non-selective. It is quite possible that agents blocking selectively the M_3 receptors or at least not affecting M_2 receptors might be more potent anticholinergic bronchodilators. Tiotropium, a new long-acting preparation binds to all three receptor subtypes, but it has a duration of action up to 10 times longer at M_3 than M_2.[8]

There have been many arguments over the effectiveness of β-agonists and anticholinergic bronchodilators in COPD. Both can be effective bronchodilators. β-agonists have a faster onset of action and ipratropium lasts a little longer than short acting β-agonists, but not so long as the long-acting β-agonists. At low doses, the effect may be submaximal such that a second drug or the combination may provide an additional benefit. At maximally effective doses, there is evidence in some studies for a greater effect from ipratropium

bromide. The results are variable, if anything anticholinergic agents have a slightly greater effect.

Some studies suggest that age may be related to the different responses to β-agonists and anticholinergic drugs. Whereas β-agonist receptors become less effective with time, the anticholinergic response is maintained, thus increasing the relative effectiveness of anticholinergic drugs in older patients.

Oxitropium bromide appears to have a slightly longer action than ipratropium bromide but any differences are slight. In contrast, tiotropium has shown a much more prolonged bronchodilation, and appears to be an effective once daily bronchidilator (Fig. 6.6). Trials involving other measures of effect such as health status and sleep quality are in progress.

Possible adverse effects of the anticholinergic drugs are:

- Dry mouth;
- Urinary retention;
- Glaucoma;
- Constipation;
- Drying of secretions.

At normal doses, none of these are a problem although precipitation of glaucoma has been recorded and measurements of intraocular pressure show a small rise. When a nebulizer is used there is the potential for a loose-fitting

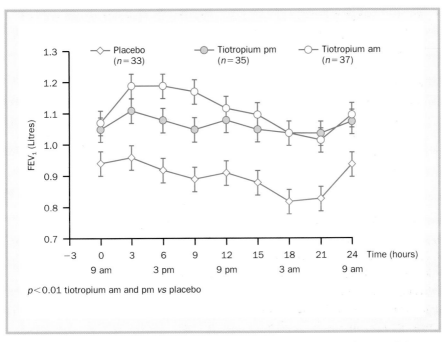

Figure 6.6
Tiotropium am/pm dosing: improvement in FEV$_1$ over 24 hours (at steady rate). (Adapted from Calverley et al[8]).

mask to direct some of the drug directly into the eye and cause pupillary dilatation.

Delivery of inhaled bronchodilators

Patients with COPD may have particular problems with the use of drugs by inhalation. Some studies have shown increased problems of co-ordination with metered-dose inhalers in the elderly. Other conditions such as arthritis

may make some devices difficult to use, and dose counters on some devices may be difficult for those with limited vision. In addition, the low inspiratory flow rates achievable in severe COPD may be insufficient for some of the dry-powder devices. Therefore particular attention needs to be paid to the use of drugs by inhalation in COPD. The technique should be checked regularly.

With the variety of inhaler devices

available, the majority of patients with COPD can be given their bronchodilators by this route. It may require some time finding the most suitable device and individuals may be best suited to a spacer attachment, a breath-actuated device or a dry-powder system. Home nebulizers have been used widely for bronchodilator therapy in COPD. One of the advantages of nebulizers is that they are able to deliver a high dose more conveniently than by multiple administration of an inhaler. The majority of COPD patients, however, do not benefit greatly from a dose above two to four puffs of a standard metered-dose inhaler. In some patients, the delivery of the greater volume of the nebulisate and the

bronchodilator may help sputum clearance (Fig. 6.7).

In addition nebulizers may be helpful during acute exacerbations when reduced flow rates and coughing may limit inhaler use. Some studies have shown that an inhaler and spacer device can substitute for a nebulizer in acute exacerbations.

The use of home nebulizers is an expensive option, not only because of the initial investment in the machine but the cost of the nebulized drug solutions and the provision of a maintenance programme to service machines.

When nebulizers are being considered for home use they should be evaluated carefully

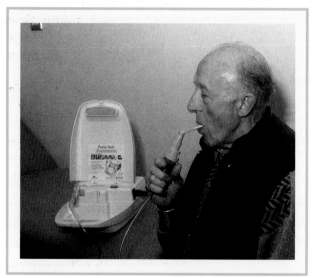

Figure 6.7
Nebulizers provide a convenient way of delivering large doses of drug but the same effect can often be produced by simpler delivery devices.

and the patient should be assessed by a respiratory physician. The British Thoracic Society guidelines[9] on '*Current Best Practice for Nebuliser Treatment*' have suggested a series of steps in the assessment for home nebulizers:

1. Assess response to a hand held inhaler selected for the particular patient;
2. Assess response to 2 weeks' oral or high-dose inhaled steroids;
3. Assess responses to higher doses by inhalation;
4. If response is poor, assess nebulizer effect at home for 2 weeks with peak flow and symptom monitoring;
5. If peak flow response is >15% then need for home nebulizer depends on clinical judgement;
6. One off reversibility tests may not predict subsequent responses;
7. Advise use up to four times daily;
8. Review regularly in respiratory clinic.

These are stringent recommendations. In practice, the clinical judgement of the clinician is very important in deciding to embark on a trial of nebulizer use and in assessing the response. Peak flow is not an ideal assessment of effect in COPD, and removing a nebulizer from a patient who thinks it is useful may be difficult.

Methylxanthines

Methylxanthines have been used for hundreds of years as bronchodilators, currently theophylline is the main form in use. When given intravenously the ethylenediamine salt aminophylline is used. The mechanism of action is still poorly understood, although the 'traditional explanation' is that inhibition of phosphodiesterase, leads to an increase in intracellular cyclic AMP but other, better phosphodiesterase inhibitors have less effect. Other effects on respiratory muscle strength and fatigue, increasing diaphragmatic action, have been proposed but are disputed at usual drug levels.

The position of theophylline has changed markedly over the last 30 years from a first-line drug in COPD to a third-line one after β-agonists and anticholinergic bronchodilators. A major reason for this change is the use of the inhaled route for the other drugs, limiting their toxicity. In contrast, adverse effects of methylxanthines are a significant problem. The clearance of theophylline varies significantly between individuals. It also decreases with age and is significantly affected by other drugs and conditions.

Sustained-release preparations allow better profiles of drug levels and easier control. However, drug levels should be monitored about 1 week after changes in dose and at regular intervals. This should be every 6–12 months in COPD to deal with changes in

Table 6.2 Factors affecting theophylline metabolism in COPD

Reduced clearance	Increased clearance
• Erythromycin	• Cigarette smoking
• Cimetidine	• Phenytoin therapy
• Ciprofloxacin	• Alcohol
• Allopurinol	
• Frusemide	
• Cirrhosis	
• Cardiac failure	
• Cor pulmonale	
• Sustained fever	
• Age	
• Influenza vaccine	

cardiac, renal and liver function, and serves as a check on compliance. In addition, care should be taken using any of the drugs in the table that interact or when the conditions also listed in the table are present.

Given all these caveats, theophylline remains a useful drug in COPD. Several studies have looked at the benefit in COPD irreversible on spirometry or in patients already taking inhaled bronchodilators. Some of these studies have shown a benefit in terms of spirometry, lung deflation, walking distance or symptomatic benefit. The current guidelines, however, all place theophylline as the third choice of the bronchodilators in COPD. It should be considered for a trial of its subjective and objective benefit in patients who are still symptomatic when using β-agonists and anticholinergics. The dose should

be increased until blood levels of 10–20 mg/l are reached. Within this range, a significant number of patients will suffer gastrointestinal side-effects but the more serious problems of arrhythmias and fits are rare.

Bronchodilators in acute exacerbations

The place of bronchodilators in acute exacerbations is dealt with in Chapter 9. They are an important part of the treatment of acute exacerbations. In general, the same principles apply of treatment by inhaled therapy, using nebulizers if necessary. In severe exacerbations not responding to other therapy, intravenous aminophylline might be considered. Care will need to be taken if the patient is already receiving oral theophylline.

New bronchodilators

Several new possibilities in bronchodilator therapy for COPD are emerging. Mention has already been made of tiotropium with its long duration of action at the M_3 receptor, providing 24 hour bronchodilation. Further advances in selectivity for M_1 and M_3 receptors may improve the effectiveness of anticholinergic agents.

In the area of methylxanthines there is growing interest in selective phosphodiesterase inhibitors, which show anti-inflammatory and bronchodilatory characteristics, without the complications of receptor down-regulation and increased bronchial reactivity. Seven families of PDE isoenzymes have been isolated. PDE_{IV} inhibitors have shown promising results and are the subject of clinical trials. The results for second-generation compounds have been encouraging.

A rational approach to bronchodilator use in COPD

Bronchodilators are used for symptomatic relief. In mild COPD this may mean occasional use but, in moderate COPD, the symptoms are not usually completely relieved by treatment. The need is, therefore, for regular treatment with additional therapy when needed. β-Agonists and anticholinergics seem to produce broadly similar effects so either can be used first line with a combination as needs increase. Combining drugs may produce fewer adverse effects than a higher dose of a single drug, although side-effects with inhaled therapy are uncommon. The existence of long-acting drugs suggests the best approach may be to use these regularly with a shorter-acting agent as needed. If this still proves inadequate after checking inhaler technique and compliance a trial of theophylline should be considered.

Practical points

- Inhaled bronchodilators form a major part of the treatment of COPD;
- Bronchodilators are administered usually by inhaled devices;
- Careful attention must be paid to inhaler technique in COPD patients;
- Nebulisers are useful for some severe cases but should be evaluated carefully;
- Anticholinergic bronchodilators produce as good or better responses than beta agonists;
- Long-acting inhaled beta agonists have been shown to produce significant improvement in symptoms and quality of life;
- Long-acting inhaled anticholinergics such as tiotropium may provide benefit from once daily inhalation;
- Theophylline is an effective bronchodilator but associated with more side effects than inhaled therapy.

References

1   Oga T, Nishimura K, Tsukino M, et al. The effects of oxitropium bromide on exercise performance in patients with stable chronic obstructive pulmonary disease. A comparison of three different exercise tests. *Am J Respir Crit Care Med* 2000;**161**:1897–901.

2   Wegner RE, Jorres RA, Kirsten DK, et al. Factor analysis of exercise capacity, dyspnoea ratings and lung function in patients with severe COPD. *Eur Respir J* 1994;**7**:725–9.

3   Calverley PMA. The future for tiotropium. *Chest* 2000;**117**:67S–69S.

4   Combivent Inhalation Study Group. In chronic obstructive pulmonary disease, a combination of ipatropium and albuterol is more effective than either agent alone: an 85-day multicenter trial. *Chest* 1994;**105**:1411–19.

5   Anthonisen NR, Connett JE, Kiley JP, et al. Effects of smoking intervention and the use of an inhaled anticholinergic bronchodilator on the rate of decline of FEV$_1$: the Lung Health Study. *J Am Med Assoc* 1994;**272**:1497–505.

6   van Noord JA, de Munck DR, Bantje TA, et al. Long-term treatment of chronic obstructive pulmonary disease with salmeterol and the additive effect of ipratropium. *Eur Respir J* 2000;**15**:878–85.

7   Jones PW, Bosh TK. Quality of life changes in COPD patients treated with salmeterol. *Am J Resp Crit Care Med* 1997;**155**:1283–9.

8   Calverley PMA, Towse LJ, Lee A. The timing of dose and pattern of bronchodilatation of tiotropium (TIO) in stable COPD. *Eur Respir J* 2000;**16**(Suppl 31):56s.

9   British Thoracic Society Standards of Care Committee. Current best practice for nebuliser treatment. *Thorax* 1997;**52**(Suppl 2):S1–S106.

Infection, antibiotics and vaccination

7

Introduction

Infections are the most common precipitant of exacerbations in COPD. However, infectious agents are often found in respiratory tract secretions, both *during* and *in between* exacerbations of COPD. The increased mucus production in COPD and the poorer mucociliary clearance make it more difficult to clear micro-organisms from the respiratory tract.

There has been some disagreement whether acute infective exacerbations play a role in accelerating lung damage and affect the natural history of COPD. The early studies of Fletcher et al[1] suggested that they did not affect the rate of decline of loss of lung function but some more recent studies[2] suggest a contribution with frequent infections. Infectious exacerbations certainly cause inconvenience, time off work and, in severe COPD, they may be fatal.

Some important questions that need to be addressed are:

- What infectious agents are important in COPD?
- Do anti-infectious agents help during exacerbations, if so what is the best choice?
- Is there any benefit from treatment with anti-infectious agents outside exacerbations?

- Do any vaccinations or other modulators of immune function help?

Exacerbation rates are quite variable. In several recent studies of COPD patients, such as those on inhaled corticosteroid treatment, the average number of exacerbations in moderately severe COPD was around 1.5 per year. Although severe exacerbations with fever, increased cough, productive of greater volumes of more purulent sputum may be obvious, there has been some difficulty in obtaining an easily applied definition of exacerbations. The most frequently used definition is the presence of two or more of the following:

1. Increased breathlessness;
2. Increased sputum production;
3. Development of purulent sputum.

With this definition, antibiotics have been shown to be useful in management of infection in COPD.

Infectious agents in exacerbations of COPD

Information about the infective agent in COPD comes usually from sputum culture. However, the sputum may be contaminated as it passes through the upper airways. It is possible to obtain samples directly from the lower respiratory tract using protected brushes within a casing with a wax plug. The brush is introduced through a bronchoscope and pushed out of its protective layer once in the lower airways. This can be used to explore the microbiology of the bronchial tree but is not a practical technique to obtain material to guide treatment. Such studies show that the lower airways may be colonized in COPD and more bacteria are isolated during exacerbations.

The organisms isolated most often, in about equal proportions, are:

- *Streptococcus pneumoniae*;
- *Haemophilus influenzae*;
- *Moraxella cattarrhalis*;
- Viruses especially rhinoviruses.

Antibiotics in acute exacerbations

When patients present with acute exacerbations it is important to rule out important differential diagnoses such as pneumonia and pneumothorax. Most published studies of antibiotics in acute exacerbations of COPD represent trials comparing a new antibiotic with a standard drug. Many such trials continue to be published but most are too small to show a difference or to demonstrate equivalence of drugs. Only a minority of trials have compared an antibiotic with placebo. These were included in a meta-analysis published in 1995.[3] This study found nine adequate, randomized, placebo-controlled trials. Four trials were conducted on in-patients. The main conclusion was that antibiotics were significantly better than placebo but only by a little. Days of symptoms were marginally shorter. Peak flow rates recovered slightly more quickly (mean 11 litres/minute) particularly in those more impaired to start. This analysis backs up the use of antibiotics in COPD, particularly in severe exacerbations but shows that the effects are not dramatic; patients with mild exacerbations will recover even without antibiotics. These results apply to acute exacerbations of COPD. Similar studies in acute bronchitis without underlying COPD show no significant benefit from antibiotics.

Anecdotal accounts suggest that, if an antibiotic is to be used then the sooner it is used the better. This means that it may be useful to encourage patients to hold a supply of antibiotics at home and to educate them to use them when their symptoms meet the criteria of an acute exacerbation, that is, when their sputum has increased significantly in volume and purulence or their breathlessness has increased with a change in sputum. This avoids the delays in the system where patients develop symptoms, have to feel ill enough to make an appointment, get their prescription and then take it to a pharmacist for their antibiotics. If patients keep the drug at home they can start taking the course and make an appointment to check that they are

responding, to review whether the course of action was appropriate and to collect a further antibiotic course for next time.

Prophylactic antibiotics, however, are not thought to be helpful in most patients. It may be that they should be considered in the occasional patients with very frequent infective exacerbations, particularly over the winter months. Very frequent infective exacerbations might also prompt a search for underlying bronchiectasis using high-resolution CT scan in a few patients.

Choice of antibiotic

The usual sensitivities of the three common bacteria are shown in Table 7.1. There will be local differences in the pattern of resistance of these organisms. In practice, it seems that the particular antibiotic choice is not crucial. Most of the common broadly acting agents are effective and it is useful to follow local guidelines based on sensitivities of local isolates. Common choices are amoxycillin, amoxycillin/clavulinic acid, doxycycline. There is no indication to use newer, more expensive agents or to cover a wider range of organisms in acute exacerbations of COPD.

Common side-effects of common antibiotics used are shown in Table 7.2.

Table 7.1
Sensitivities of three common bacteria to antibiotics

Antibiotic	S. pneumoniae	H. influenzae	M. catarrhalis
Amoxycillin	+	+/−	−
Amoxycillin/clavulinic acid	+	+	+
Doxycycline	+/−	+/−	+
Erythromycin	+	+/−	+
Trimethoprim	+/−	+?	+?
Clarithromycin/azithromycin	+	+/−	+
Cefaclor	+/−	+/−	+/−

+, sensitive; −, resistant; +/−, partially sensitive.

Table 7.2
Common side-effects of current antibiotics used in COPD

Antibiotic	Common adverse effects
Amoxycillin	Hypersensitivity reactions, gastrointestinal upset
Amoxycillin/clavulinic acid	Hypersensitivity reactions, gastrointestinal upset, hepatic toxicity
Doxycycline	Gastrointestinal disturbance, photosensitivity, allergic reactions, oesophagitis
Erythromycin	Gastrointestinal disturbance, cholestatic jaundice, allergic reactions
Trimethoprim	Gastrointestinal disturbance, skin rashes, folate deficiency
Clarithromycin/azithromycin	Gastrointestinal disturbance, hepatic dysfunction, allergic reactions
Cefaclor	Hypersensitivity reactions, gastrointestinal upset

Influenza immunization

Epidemics of influenza cause a significant mortality in patients with COPD. Most COPD guidelines recommend the use of influenza vaccination annually. The usual vaccine is a killed vaccine. They are trivalent (two subtypes of influenza A and one of B). The virus strains are chosen according to virulence, lack of community immunity, predicted strains and ability to culture. The combination is developed and tested over 6 months and available from around October. Immunization remains the most effective way of protecting against influenza. It is regarded as appropriate for all patients with COPD and other chronic respiratory disorders on an annual basis. Although effectiveness has been demonstrated in young and older populations there is no evidence specific to COPD. In young, healthy populations protection is around 70% with suitable vaccines. In the elderly, the response is less but hospitalizations are reduced by about 50% and mortality of influenza epidemics reduced even though cases of influenza are only decreased by 30–40%.

The immunization in adults consists of 0.5 ml given by intramuscular or deep subcutaneous injection over the deltoid muscle. It can be given at the same time as pneumococcal vaccination but at a different site. Influenza vaccination should not be given in the presence of an acute febrile illness. It should also be avoided in patients known to be allergic to eggs or poultry. Cases of Guillain-Barré syndrome have been reported; however, this is rare — estimated to be 1–2 per million. Patients often report a short febrile episode but influenza itself cannot be related to a killed virus. In the future, a live attenuated intranasal virus may become available.

In patients who cannot receive influenza vaccination because of anaphylaxis associated with eggs, prophylaxis with amantadine should be considered in high-risk situations.

Zanamavir: a new anti-viral drug

Zanamavir is from a new class of drugs with better efficiency and less toxicity than existing anti-viral drugs. It acts as a competitive inhibitor of influenza A and B virus neurominidase. Administration is by inhalation 10 mg twice daily, started as soon as possible in the infection. There have been anxieties in the UK about the lack of evidence specific to older patients, particularly with COPD, and further studies are underway.

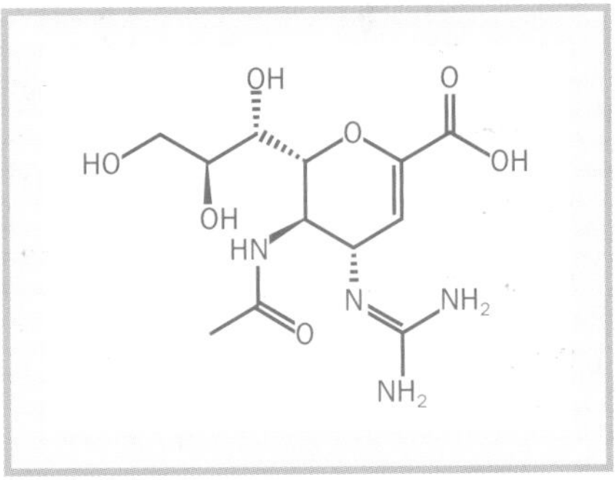

Figure 7.1
Neuraminidase is a glycoprotein projecting from the surface of influenza viruses. It breaks the bond linking flu virus particles to the cell allowing spread of infection. Neuraminidase inhibitors such as zanamivir prevent this release and reduce symptoms if given within 36 hours of onset of confirmed influenza.

Available studies, however, show a reduction in illness of up to 2.5 days.[4] Potentially this may be very beneficial. Practical difficulties include the ability to deliver the drug early enough in episodes of influenza and the need to avoid delivery to patients with another mild upper respiratory infection rather than influenza. It would seem sensible, at present, to consider zanamavir in patients with underlying COPD becoming unwell with typical symptoms during an influenza epidemic. Care is needed to ensure patients can cope with the inhaler device.

Pneumococcal vaccination

The 23 valent vaccine contains polysaccharides from 23 of the most common and virulent serotypes. Results of good trials in COPD do not yet exist. By extrapolation from other situations and the knowledge that *Streptococcus pneumoniae* is a pathogen have led to its use in COPD. The pneumococcal vaccine should certainly be considered in patients with frequent exacerbations. It can be given at the same time as influenza virus and does not need to be repeated for at least 5–6 years.

Pneumococcal vaccination is given in a volume of 0.5 ml intramuscularly or subcutaneously. Low-grade fever and local reactions can occur.

Non-specific immune system modulation

Broncho-Vaxom is a mixture of bacterial products intended to stimulate immune responses by way of macrophages. It has been reported to reduce the severity of exacerbations. At present it is not available in the UK.

Practical approach

In moderately severe COPD, the treatment regime for infective elements might be as follows:

- Annual influenza vaccination;
- Course of antibiotic (amoxycillin or doxycycline to keep at home and start for 7 days at the onset of an exacerbation);
- Pneumococcal vaccination every 5 years if exacerbations frequent (>2 significant exacerbations per year);
- Consider high resolution CT scan and/or course of 2–3 months of antibiotic if over four exacerbations per year.

Practical points

- The most common organisms in exacerbations are viruses, Streptococcus pneumoniae, Haemophilus influenzae, and Moraxella cattarrhalis;
- Antibiotics in acute exacerbations produce results slightly but significantly better than placebo;

- Simple cheap antibiotics are appropriate for most patients;
- Annual influenza vaccination is recommended in COPD;
- Zanamavir reduces the length of an episode of influenza if started within 36 hours of the onset of symptoms;
- Pneumococcal vaccination may be of benefit for patients with COPD;
- Pneumococcal vaccination does not need to be repeated for at least 5–6 years.

References

1   Fletcher C, Peto R. The natural history of chronic airflow obstruction. *Br Med J* 1977;1:1645–8.

2   Burge PS, Calverley PM, Jones PW, et al. Randomised, double blind, placebo controlled study of fluticasone propionate in patients with moderate to severe chronic obstructive pulmonary disease: the ISOLDE trial. *BMJ* 2000;**320**:1297–303.

3   Saint S, Bent S, Vittinghoff E, Grady D. Antibiotics in chronic obstructive pulmonary disease exacerbations. A meta-analysis. *J Am Med Assoc* 1995;**273**: 957–60.

4   Silagy CA, Campion C. Effectiveness and role of zanamavir in the treatment of influenza infection. *Ann Med* 1999;**31**:313–17.

Anti-inflammatory therapy

8

Introduction

Given the central importance of inflammation as the underlying mechanism of COPD, it is not surprising that attempts to suppress this by medical means have been studied widely. For a long time there was considerable confusion about who and when to treat, a problem that has still not been completely resolved with the publication of a series of longer-term studies of inhaled corticosteroids in the last few years. The decision to prescribe this therapy is one of the more contentious that the physician has to make in the area of COPD care, and so this chapter will try to summarize what we know presently with any certainty and suggest an approach that may help with this decision in practice.

Types of inflammatory therapy

The characteristics of the inflammatory change in COPD have been reviewed in Chapter 2. It is clear that this is not an allergy-driven process and so it is not surprising that therapies used to modify allergic inflammation have little role here. Occasional studies of disodium cromoglycate and nedocromil in small numbers of COPD patients have shown no benefit, and these drugs are not indicated in COPD management. On first principles, it is unlikely that the leukotriene antagonists will be particularly helpful but there are virtually no data about the generation of leukotrienes in COPD, and no clinical studies have been reported. One leukotriene, LTB4, is known to be generated by a non-cyclo-oxygenase-dependent mechanism in exacerbations of COPD. This is a potent leucocyte chemoattractant, and specific antagonists have been developed and they are currently undergoing clinical trials. Whether they prove effective will depend on the importance of this mediator in neutrophil recruitment, and also the ability of the drug to reach the airway in sufficient amounts after being given orally.

Much the most studied anti-inflammatory drugs are the corticosteroids, which are potent and relatively non-specific anti-inflammatory agents. Several mechanisms for their anti-inflammatory action have been proposed. There is evidence for nuclear transcription of specific glucocorticoid responsive elements that prevent the synthesis of proinflammatory cytokines and nitric oxide. Recently, there has been interest in the effect of glucocorticoids on the extranuclear transcription factor NFκB, which may explain why sometimes they can produce effects more quickly than anticipated from a purely nuclear action.

These anti-inflammatory effects are relatively non-specific and occur in diseases where CD4$^+$ lymphocytes predominate, as in bronchial asthma, and in others where CD8$^+$ cells are important, like rheumatoid arthritis. There is increasing evidence, however, that cigarette smoking can block the effects of corticosteroids in asthma, and perhaps in COPD. This may be due to a specific blocking action at the NFκB level or an effect on the mechanism responsible for allowing the corticosteroid access to the nuclear chromatin. Further elucidation of this potentially important mechanism is awaited.

Experimental studies

These have only begun in earnest recently, and have produced a range of conflicting results depending on the endpoint adopted. Early studies with inhaled beclomethasone suggested that the degree of inflammation scored visually was reduced by the inhaled drug, as was the amount of protein leak.[1] Studies of the short-term effects of inhaled fluticasone on sputum elastolytic activity suggested that this could be reduced with the active drug.[2] The number of neutrophils present in induced sputum was reduced by inhaled corticosteroids in one study but a series of carefully conducted experiments from the National Heart and Lung Institute found no effect of corticosteroids whether oral or inhaled on a range of inflammatory markers in induced sputum including TNFα and IL-8.[3]

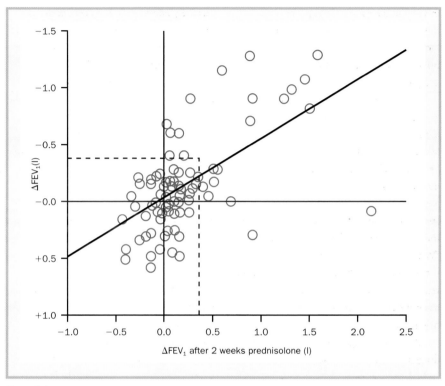

Figure 8.1
Improvements in spirometry in patients identified as responding to oral corticosteroids. All patients were treated with inhaled steroids and those with the largest initial responses tended to show most improvement at one year. Modified with permission from Davies et al.[4]

Biopsy studies are much more limited but one investigation found no effect on the major cell populations but a reduction in mast cell numbers after corticosteroid therapy. This differs significantly from the position in asthma where substantial changes in biopsy appearances occur after any form of corticosteroid treatment.

Identifying susceptible subjects

This is often performed by conducting a trial of corticosteroid treatment either oral or inhaled. Practical details of this are given in Chapter 3. The best validated outcome measure is a change in the FEV_1 but, given the between-day reproducibility of this measurement of approximately 200 ml and change between measurements made several weeks apart, this change needs to exceed 400 ml before it can be attributed to the treatment rather than being a chance finding. Studies of groups of patients reduces this variation but, for the individual patient, an increase in FEV_1 of 300 ml is not necessarily a pointer to future long-term improvement.[5] Patients who appear to respond can be identified by prior bronchodilator testing, where a large response will select patients who continue to improve after inhaled corticosteroids (Fig. 8.1).[4] Small changes in FEV_1 after an oral trial of treatment usually exhibit regression to the mean with time. Despite these caveats, a few patients with a positive corticosteroid trial, will have clinically worthwhile benefits after inhaled steroids. These are more likely to be found among the more severe patients. These patients do not have asthmatic features and cannot be identified by simple clinical or laboratory testing. One study has suggested that increased eosinophil numbers in induced sputum from these patients are predictive of a physiological or symptomatic response; however, larger studies will be needed to validate this approach. Even after successful oral and inhaled therapy these patients still have features of clinically important airflow obstruction.

Among patients with very limited or absent bronchodilator responsiveness, the results of an oral steroid trial are very disappointing. Individuals thought to be responsive were no more or less likely to have a subsequent accelerated loss of lung function or to have frequent exacerbations. In one large study, however, the absolute size of the change in FEV_1 after oral prednisolone for 2 weeks was significantly less in those who smoked.

Early clinical studies

Although a wide range of clinical endpoints have been considered, the most important hypothesis to be tested was that regular corticosteroid therapy can return the rate of decline of FEV_1 towards normal levels. Assessing this requires careful methodology and patient selection, as well as involving large numbers of patients followed over several years. Before this occurred, several studies of different populations were undertaken that tended to support the view that corticosteroid therapy was having an effect on the rate of decline of FEV_1.

The earliest observations came from The Netherlands where a retrospective analysis suggested that patients treated with oral corticosteroids included a subset who showed temporary improvement in lung function before declining again. A subsequent report claimed that regular inhaled corticosteroids (ICS) produced significant increases in baseline FEV_1 over 21 months. The difficulty was that most of these patients were found on a retrospective review to be asthmatic.[6] More promising was the report by Dompeling and colleagues that introducing inhaled corticosteroid to patients known to show a decline in lung function could reduce that decline,[7] a finding subsequently supported by a meta-analysis of several randomized controlled trials of budesonide and beclomethasone in COPD. Paggiaro and co-workers studied a large number of moderately severe patients over 6 months and found that those treated with inhaled fluticasone had better exercise performance and fewer exacerbations than the control patients.[8] An uncontrolled observational study noted that withdrawing inhaled corticosteroids led to an increase in exacerbations in patients who were previously stable. All of these studies suggested that some form of biological effect was present, although the magnitude of this and its nature were unclear. This situation has improved somewhat with the publication of several larger and longer trials of ICS therapy in several different patient groups. The principal outcome of these trials is shown in Figure 8.2

Major treatment trials

All of these studies were double-blind, placebo-controlled and randomized. All followed the patients over 3 years, selected patients with almost no evidence of bronchodilator responsiveness and used the same particularly rigorous method of statistical analysis. This similarity in design allows us to combine their data (Fig. 8.3) but, even in these very similar studies, there are

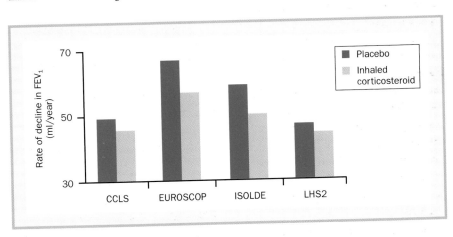

Figure 8.2
Rate of decline in FEV_1 for placebo and inhaled corticosteroid groups in four large trials.

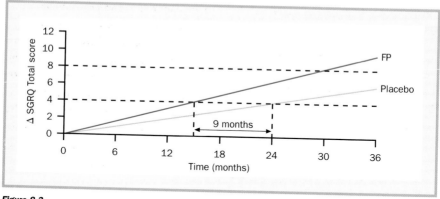

Figure 8.3
Decline in health status was slower on fluticasone than placebo in the ISOLDE study. A change of 4 in the score is regarded as significant.

important differences that have implications for clinical practice.

The Copenhagen City Lung Study[9]

This is the smallest of the large studies and recruited from a cohort of patients identified by community survey as showing airflow obstruction with an FEV_1/FVC ratio less than 70%. Patients received budesonide 1200 µg for 6 months and then 800 µg daily thereafter. Pulmonary function assessed by FEV_1 was only slightly impaired at baseline (88% predicted post-bronchodilator therapy) and was unaffected by the active treatment, which did not modify the rate of decline in FEV_1.

The European Respiratory Society study of Chronic Obstructive Pulmonary disease (EUROSCOP)[10]

This study recruited a large number of participants from 18 European countries by advertising campaigns and having excluded those who were able to stop smoking followed the post-bronchodilator FEV_1 at 3-monthly intervals while the subjects received 800 µg budesonide or placebo. These patients were a little more severe (post-bronchodilator FEV_1 was 79% predicted) but still had relatively early disease. After 3–6 months there was a small (50 ml) increase in FEV_1 in the treated patients, which persisted throughout the trial but the rate of decline in FEV_1 was unchanged.

The Inhaled Steroids in Obstructive Lung DiseasE study (ISOLDE)[11]

Here patients were recruited from hospital outpatient clinics and could enter whether they had quit smoking or not. They were clinically and physiologically more severe (post-bronchodilator FEV_1 was 50% predicted) and most underwent an oral corticosteroid trial at the outset. They received either 1 mg of fluticasone or placebo daily and in this study two other outcomes, apart from FEV_1, were included — the number of exacerbations requiring treatment and the health status measured by the St George's Respiratory Questionnaire. Like the EUROSCOP study, there was a small but sustained increase in FEV_1 in the steroid-treated limb but no difference in the rate of decline of FEV_1. In this study, there were more drop-outs in the placebo limb of the trial mainly due to exacerbations. There was a 25% reduction in these in the treated patients who also showed a significant slowing in the decline in health status (Fig. 8.3). This is thought mainly to reflect the lower number of exacerbations in the treated group.

Lung Health Study 2

One further study is due to be published soon, the Lung Health Study 2 but details about the specific findings are not generally available at the time of writing. This is a large

study comparing triamcinolone acetonide with placebo in patients with a severity intermediate to EUROSCOP and ISOLDE. Unfortunately this drug needs to be used four times daily and not twice daily as in the other studies (where compliance was approximately 85%). In this study compliance was only 50% and, unsurprisingly, there was no effect on the rate of decline of FEV_1. Further analysis on a per protocol basis is awaited.

Side-effects and toxicity

Corticosteroids have a formidable range of toxic effects, which are summarized in Table 8.1. Most of these are well-known but particular mention should be made of the proximal myopathy, which is not often specifically sought but was frequently found in patients receiving 4 mg or more of prednisolone per day. Not only does this reduce exercise capacity but it is associated with an increased mortality. In these circumstances, given the existence of co-morbidities likely to be made overt by or interact with these numerous side-effects, there can be no place for maintenance oral corticosteroids in the care of the COPD patient.

Inhaled corticosteroids involve the use of much smaller doses and even less of these is available systemically. Nonetheless, the clinical trials mentioned indicate that some side-effects are reasonably common. Although

Table 8.1
Side effects of corticosteroids

- Central obesity, moon-face, 'buffalo hump'
- Striae, thinning of skin
- Spontaneous bruising*
- Glucose intolerance, diabetes mellitus
- Osteoporosis
- Avascular necrosis
- Fluid retention
- Peptic ulceration, GI bleeding
- Cataracts
- Peripheral muscle myopathy
- Adrenal suppression
- Pharyngeal candidiasis*
- Dysphonia*

*Documented to occur with inhaled corticosteroids

the Copenhagen[9] and EUROSCOP[10] studies used a dry-powder device (Turbohaler®), and the ISOLDE study[11] used a spacer, local complications such as oral candidiasis and hoarse voice were slightly more common in the corticosteroid treated patients. Clearly some of these drugs reached the systemic circulation, since the percentage of patients with spontaneous bruising was higher in the treated groups and measurements of morning cortisols were statistically, but not clinically, significantly reduced in the ISOLDE study. Studies of bone density in the EUROSCOP study were reassuringly normal but data from the Lung Health Study 2 suggests that some patients may lose bone mass more quickly. One of the confounding factors, particularly

in patients with more severe disease is the use of oral corticosteroids to treat exacerbations. Experience in asthma suggests that this has a much greater effect on bone metabolism than even quite prolonged inhaled steroid use.

Towards a policy for the use of inhaled corticosteroids (ICS)

These complex investigations have left clinicians with a series of rather mixed messages and a feeling of confusion, which the efforts of the pharmaceutical industry are likely to make worse. Interpretation of the present evidence should take account of several facts:

- The type of patients studied: only those in the ISOLDE study were part of the health care system; all the others were acquired by community survey or a request to join a smoking-cessation scheme. This helps separate people who might come forward from health-screening initiatives from those presenting with symptoms. Only the ISOLDE patients were sick enough for exacerbations and decline in health status to be measurable;

- The doses given are all relatively large and this is based on data in previous studies rather poorly conducted. More data is needed about whether lower doses of ICS are effective;

- The type of delivery device produced

similar satisfactory levels of compliance and broadly similar systemic side-effects. Whether targeting for less alveolar deposition is practical is unknown; on present evidence this is unlikely to have made much difference;

- The evidence that some drug is systemically available raises fears about unquantifiable side-effects, such as accelerated osteoporosis. The confounding effect of oral corticosteroids has already been mentioned but many other factors such as smoking status, gender, mobility and nutritional state complicate the interpretation of bone density measurements in this group; thus very large prospective studies will be needed to determine whether there is a real or just an imagined hazard to COPD patients of ICS;

- All of these studies included patients with minimal bronchodilator reversibility, and many patients who just fell outside of these rigid criteria were excluded from the study. Perhaps it is no surprise to find that when you study a group of patients with no variability in their FEV_1 it is very difficult to change this outcome variable. More information is needed on those patients with more labile airways disease who nonetheless meet the definition of COPD.

Despite these problems some practical conclusions can be drawn:

1. There is no evidence that ICS influence the rate of decline in FEV_1 at any stage of the illness (Fig. 8.2);

2. Since patients with mild or asymptomatic disease are unlikely to benefit and, being younger, would be exposed to any side-effects for longer, ICS should not be offered to these patients;

3. Patients with established disease who show a substantial bronchodilator response merit a therapeutic trial of oral or inhaled corticosteroid. Failure to maintain this benefit if the treatment has been used regularly is an indication to discontinue this treatment;

4. Patients who do not have a large bronchodilator response or where this information is not available may still show benefits in terms of reduced exacerbations and improved well being if their baseline FEV_1 is less than 1.5 l (based on the ISOLDE[11] and Paggiarro[8] data). This benefit is likely to be greatest if they have had an exacerbation severe enough to merit oral corticosteroid therapy in the last year;

5. Where the concern about side-effects is high or the initial indication for therapy is weak, patients can stop ICS. It is prudent, however, to withdraw treatment over a couple of weeks to reduce the chance of precipitating an exacerbation.

The future

Whatever their present role in COPD care, it is clear that use of ICS alone is ineffective in controlling disease progression. Studies are already underway to determine whether long-acting beta-agonists alone or in combination with ICS can produce better control of exacerbation and improve health status. As noted in Chapter 1, antioxidants have the potential to be effective anti-inflammatory drugs, and a new more potent derivative of *N* acetyl cysteine is being developed to test this possibility. The early promise of neutrophil elastase inhibitors appears limited by their toxic effects. The most promising agent currently in clinical trials is a phosphodiesterase 4 inhibitor, which has a good anti-inflammatory profile and a much more acceptable side-effect profile compared with non-specific phosphodiesterase inhibitors like theophylline. Even if the early encouraging results are confirmed in larger studies there is still much time-consuming clinical work to undertake before this or any other agent can be considered to have a disease-modifying effect in COPD. The development of simple exhaled breath tests, which can measure the inflammatory status of the lower respiratory tract, may allow to select the best candidates from the many new agents now proposed for the anti-inflammatory treatment of COPD.

Practical points

- The inflammatory process in COPD differs from that in asthma;
- Large scale controlled trials in COPD have shown that inhaled corticosteroids make no difference to rate of decline of lung function in smokers or mixed groups of smokers and non-smokers;
- The trials in more severe patients show a reduction in exacerbations with inhaled steroids;
- Trials in more severe patients suggest a benefit on quality of life with high doses of inhaled steroids;
- Adverse effects such as bruising are increased on inhaled steroids in COPD;
- It is uncertain whether the benefits can be obtained with lower doses of inhaled corticosteroids;
- Careful attention needs to be paid to inhaler technique and compliance;
- Other agents such as antioxidants and phosphodiesterase 4 inhibitors are being studied.

References

1   Thompson AB, Mueller MB, Heires AJ, et al. Aerosolized beclomethasone in chronic bronchitis. Improved pulmonary function and diminished airway inflammation. *Am Rev Respir Dis* 1992;**146**:389–95.

2   Llewellyn-Jones CG, Harris TAJ, Stockley RA. Effect of fluticasone propionate on

sputum of patients with chronic bronchitis and emphysema. *Am J Respir Crit Care Med* 1996;**153**:616–21.

3 Keatings VM, Jatakanon A, Worsdell YM, Barnes PJ. Effects of inhaled and oral glucocorticoids on inflammatory indices in asthma and COPD. *Am J Respir Crit Care Med* 1997;**155**:542–8.

4 Davies L, Nisar M, Pearson MG, et al. Oral corticosteroid trials in the management of stable chronic obstructive pulmonary disease. *Quart J Med* 1999;**92**:395–400.

5 Nisar M, Walshaw M, Earis JE et al. Assessment of reversibility of airway obstruction in patients with chronic obstructive airways disease. *Thorax* 1990;**45**:190–4.

6 Kerstjens HA, Brand PL, Hughes MD, et al. A comparison of bronchodilator therapy with or without inhaled corticosteroid therapy for obstructive airways disease. Dutch Chronic Non-specific Lung Disease Study Group. *N Engl J Med* 1992;**327**:1413–19.

7 Dompeling E, Van Schayck CP, Van Grunsven PM, et al. Slowing the deterioration of asthma and chronic obstructive pulmonary disease observed during bronchodilator therapy by adding inhaled corticosteroids. A 4-year prospective study. *Ann Int Med* 1993;**118**:770–8.

8 Paggiaro PL, Dahle R, Bakran I, et al. Multicentre randomised placebo-controlled trial of inhaled fluticasone propionate in patients with chronic obstructive pulmonary disease. International COPD Study Group. *Lancet* 1998;**351**:773–80.

9 Vestbo J, Sorensen T, Lange P, et al. Long-term effect of inhaled budesonide in mild and moderate chronic obstructive pulmonary disease: A randomised controlled trial. *Lancet* 1999;**353**:1819–23.

10 Pauwels RA, Lofdahl C-G, Laitinen LA, et al. Long-term treatment with inhaled budesonide in persons with mild chronic obstructive pulmonary disease who continue smoking. *N Engl J Med* 1999;**340**:1948–53.

11 Burge PS, Calverley PM, Jones PW, et al. Randomised, double blind, placebo controlled study of fluticasone propionate in patients with moderate to severe chronic obstructive pulmonary disease: the ISOLDE trial. *BMJ.* 2000;**320**:1297–303.

Exacerbations of COPD

9

Introduction

Periodic worsening of the symptoms of COPD is a well-recognized part of the illness and is usually termed an *exacerbation* of COPD. Everyone seems to understand what this term means but defining it precisely can be extremely difficult.[1] As a result, there is no universally agreed definition of exactly what constitutes an exacerbation; however several general features can be stated about this process:

1. Although we talk about an exacerbation of disease there is little evidence that the underlying pathology deteriorates during these episodes. Thus there is no new or recent-onset emphysema or small airways disease precipitating new symptoms. Instead, some intercurrent insult has caused a temporary worsening of the established inflammatory process, which often results in a transient deterioration in lung mechanics and gas exchange and hence an increase in symptoms.
2. Exacerbations are symptomatic events, at least as seen clinically. Asymptomatic fluctuations in lung function without symptoms have not yet been described in COPD.

3. Exacerbations are *discrete* episodes lasting for at least 24 hours and commonly very much longer, before finally resolving. Usually 7–10 days is the average duration of an exacerbation but more detailed analysis of daily peak expiratory flow (PEF) recordings suggest that it can be 5 weeks or more before the baseline lung function is reached again after a severe episode. In sicker patients, the effect on health status can be cumulative, with the baseline level of well being never reached before the next episode supervenes. This is a potent mechanism for the progressive decline in health status that characterizes more severe COPD.

4. The severity of an exacerbation in terms of the patient's symptoms and their use of health care resources is seldom dictated by the nature of the precipitating factor but is almost entirely a consequence of the underlying severity of the COPD. Thus, although a lower respiratory tract infection with *S. pneumoniae* can lead to a few days off work and a course of antibiotics in a patient with an FEV_1 of 2.5 l. Infection with the same micro-organism can precipitate devastating respiratory failure and an ICU admission in a patient with an FEV_1 of 0.7 l. There is no evidence that the incidence of infections is higher in COPD and their IgA-mediated humeral immunity is intact; however the consequences of a 'normal' respiratory infection are more noticeable and the symptoms it produces last longer in those with COPD.

Typical symptoms seen in an exacerbation are listed in Table 9.1. These are based on the

Table 9.1
Typical symptoms, which must be present for two or more consecutive days, during an exacerbation in chronic obstructive pulmonary disorder. (After Bhowmik et al.[2])

Major Symptoms:	Increased dyspnoea Increased sputum purulence Increased sputum volume
Minor Symptoms:	Cold symptoms (nasal discharge/congestion) Sore throat Wheeze Cough Fever

An exacerbation involves two major symptoms or one major and one minor criteria of Anthonisen and colleagues[3] and have been modified on the basis of their extensive clinical data by the East London COPD group.[4] As with stable disease, cough and increasing volumes of purulent sputum are major findings in mild COPD, while worsening breathlessness despite routine therapy is the dominant and most feared symptom in those with severe disease.

The impact of exacerbations

Exacerbations of COPD are now recognized to have serious consequences for both the patient and society. Again the nature of these is dependent on the background disease severity.

For the individual

Detailed data about the effects of exacerbations in mild-to-moderate COPD (FEV_1 > 50% predicted) are lacking. It is certainly enough to cause a significant number of medical consultations for antibiotics, especially during the winter months. Indirect data suggests that chronic sputum production and cough, a marker for more frequent exacerbations, is associated with a greater number of hospitalizations for pneumonia and possibly contributes to the accelerated decline in FEV_1 that characterizes COPD.

The traditional view is that pulmonary function returns to normal after an exacerbation; whether this is still true in more severe disease when exacerbations are frequent is untested. The impact of the disease in such patients, as assessed by health status measurements, is significantly greater in those with more frequent exacerbations than those who rarely experience exacerbations. This is true even when the exacerbation does not require hospital treatment.[5] Such people are more likely to be hospitalized in future and to require more intensive medical therapy, such as wet nebulizers at home. Whether their mortality is greater than those with equivalent lung function impairment who do not experience exacerbations is unknown but appears likely to be the case.

For society

Exacerbations are one of the major drivers of health care costs in COPD. They cause significant numbers of medical consultations, which usually end in the prescription of additional therapy. Hospitalization is the single greatest component of the overall costs of COPD and acute exacerbations are the usual reason for this. In the UK direct costs of the COPD to the NHS are around £500 m. In urban areas, exacerbations of COPD are the commonest cause of respiratory hospitalization and are second only to 'chest pain' as a medical cause of admission. Numbers of admissions with exacerbations of COPD have increased significantly in recent years reflecting the ageing population and they contribute significantly to the 'winter bed pressures' that stress the UK system.

too early discharge

Aetiology

Although most episodes are precipitated by infection, this is not the only reason for an exacerbation. Several community surveys have shown that hospitalization for COPD rises in parallel with changes in atmospheric pollutants, such as ozone and nitrogen dioxide, as well as increasing significantly when the ambient temperature falls. This is likely to reflect local increases in airway inflammation rather than changes in the lung parenchyma. If exacerbations are defined in terms of deterioration in blood gas tensions rather than symptomatically, a much wider range of non-infective causes can be considered, for example pulmonary embolism and congestive cardiac failure. The clinical presentations in such cases, however, are usually sufficiently different as to avoid confusion at least in hospital practice.

Good data about the prevalence and type of infective causes of exacerbations is still surprisingly sketchy but most reports using modern virological diagnostic techniques suggest that between 35 and 40% of episodes of community-based exacerbations are associated with recent viral infection — especially with the picorna and rhinovirus groups. Influenza shows the expected

seasonality and adenoviral infection appears to be rare.[4] Secondary bacterial infection is seen in many of these cases and bacteria can be isolated in approximately 30% of cases. The presence of increased volumes of purulent sputum, especially if accompanied by worsening dyspnoea, is a strong pointer to an underlying bacterial cause.

The principal pathogens are remarkably constant year to year and are:

*   *Streptococcus pneumoniae;*
*   *Haemophilus influenzae;*
*   *Moraxella catharrhalis.*

The predominance of each varies locally and *Moraxella catharrhalis* often occurs in short-lived outbreaks and is commonly associated with a more systemic illness that is slower to resolve than the others. Other pathogens, such as coliform organisms, are only seen as nosocomial infections but may be worth considering in someone who relapses soon after discharge from hospital. The role of chronic lower respiratory tract colonization as a proof of a reservoir for these organisms is being investigated but current data suggests that it is a factor in a minority of patients.

Pathophysiology

Most information about the pathological changes during exacerbations comes from studies: (i) in relatively mild disease using bronchial biopsies; and (ii) more severe disease using induced sputum specimens. Each has its limitations but the following appears true:

- In mild disease or chronic bronchitis without airflow limitation, exacerbations are associated with increased numbers of neutrophils and eosinophils, although the latter do not reach the levels seen in bronchial asthma;
- In patients with more severe disease who have purulent sputum, neutrophils are the dominant cell type, although they are not seen in all cases;
- Elevated levels of the cytokine IL-6 have been found consistently in induced sputum from patients experiencing exacerbations, although whether this is a non-specific feature of acute inflammation or a more specific signal is unresolved. Leukotriene B4, a stimulant of neutrophil migration has been reported as being elevated in the blood of some patients;
- C-reactive protein levels are elevated for days after an acute exacerbation suggesting that a systemic effect of local airway inflammation occurs.

Physiologically, the result of this increased inflammation is to worsen airflow limitation by creating local tissue swelling, and perhaps by increasing airway smooth muscle contraction secondary to local mediator release. Increased mucus secretion from the bronchial glands contributes to local mucus plugging and sputum production, as does the increased number of neutrophils reaching the airway lumen. The cough reflex is likely to be increased by mediator release locally, and the increased mechanical burden of airway mucus which is harder to clear because it is more viscous than normal and any bacterial infection will further impair the already faulty ciliary clearance mechanisms.

The resultant worsening in lung mechanics may limit the ability to achieve normal levels of ventilation during exercise but have little further effect if the inflammation is not too severe and the overall ventilatory reserve is good. For patients with more severe disease, expiratory airflow may become limited partially or completely during tidal breathing at rest and, as a result, dynamic hyperinflation, that is an increase in end-expiratory lung volume owing to a change in breathing pattern, can occur. This can be accompanied by hyperinflation owing to complete loss of lung units and a rise in residual volume. This change in lung volume appears central to the increase in dyspnoea in these cases. It has several undesirable effects:

- It leads to intrinsic positive end-expiratory pressure (PEEPi), which must be overcome before the next breath can be initiated. This contributes substantially to the total work of breathing;
- It places the respiratory muscles at a

further geometric disadvantage and makes it harder to develop the pressure swings needed to maintain ventilation;

• It brings the respiratory muscles closer to the critical threshold where respiratory muscle fatigue develops.

The effects of these changes on gas exchange are equally important. Ventilation–perfusion mismatching worsens and hypoxaemia is an early feature in the evolution of an exacerbation, although it only becomes clinically significant in patients where hospitalization is needed. Hypercapnia occurs when the dead space ventilation increases substantially as a percentage of the tidal volume, and is associated with a rapid, shallow breathing pattern and high levels of PEEPi. Acidosis secondary to this is of considerable clinical significance (see later).

These changes are shown schematically in Fig. 9.1.

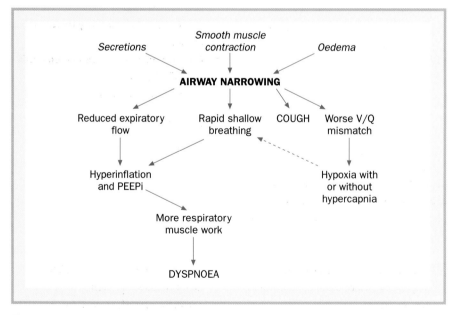

Figure 9.1
General scheme of the physiological changes occurring during exacerbations of chronic obstructive pulmonary disease. PEEPi = intrinsic positive end-expiratory pressure.

Clinical assesssment

Clinical assesssment of COPD exacerbations
depends upon the clinical setting (Table 9.2).

In the home

Clinical assessment of COPD exacerbations in the home

Look for:

Examine for:

- Recent onset of relevant symptoms
  (see Table 9.2)
- Assess level of home support
- Consider background disease severity
- History of previous hospitalization
- Presence of co-morbidities
- Current level of medical therapy

- Central cyanosis
- Respiratory rate >20/minute
- Use of accessory muscles (e.g. scalene,
  sternomastoid)
- Focal signs on auscultation/features of a
  pneumothorax
- Ankle swelling/elevated jugular venous
  pressure
- Cardiac rhythm disturbance — especially
  atrial fibrillation
- Overall level of distress

Record peak expiratory flow if possible

In the hospital

Clinical assessment of an exacerbation of
COPD in the hospital is the same as that in
the home with the addition of the following
tests:

- Measure arterial blood gases, recording the
  inspired oxygen concentration (FiO_2) if
  not on air;
- Arrange chest radiograph;
- Arrange an electrocardiogram (ECG);

- Send sputum for culture if available, and
  blood cultures if pyrexial;
- Send blood for white blood count,
  haemoglobin, urea and electrolytes as
  baseline measurements.

Managing the acute exacerbation

This involves treating the worsening airflow limitation, trying to reverse the precipitating cause (which is usually an infection) and providing appropriate physiological support until the episode spontaneously resolves. At home, this means an intensification of medical therapy, which is accompanied by other supportive treatments, for example oxygen therapy if the patient is hospitalized. Many factors contribute to a decision to send the patient to hospital (see Table 9.3) but the

most important is the lack of sufficient support in the home to manage the exacerbation there.

Mortality in COPD exacerbations is related to the presence of respiratory acidosis and other co-morbidities — particularly cardiac disease.[6] In patients with these features, 1-year survival is approximately 60% and worse still in those housebound at the time of their referral to hospital. The converse is also true, namely, that the mortality from an individual exacerbation is low in those patients hospitalized without these features. This has led several centres to develop 'home

Table 9.2
Clinical assessment of chronic obstructive pulmonary disorder exacerbations in the home.

	Treat at home	Treat in hospital
Ability to cope at home	Yes	No
Breathlessness	Mild	Severe
General condition	Good	Poor – Deteriorating
Level of activity	Good	Poor/confined to bed
Cyanosis	No	Yes
Worsening perhiperal oedema	No	Yes
Level of consciousness	Normal	Impaired
Already receiving LTOT	No	Yes
Social circumstances	Good	Living alone/not coping
Acute confusion	No	Yes
Rapid rate of onset	No	Yes
Also available at hospital		
Changes on the chest radiograph	No	Present
Arterial pH level	≥ 7.35	< 7.35
Arterial PaO$_2$	$\geq 7\,kPa$	$< 7\,kPa$

The more of the referal indicators that are present the more likely the need for admission to hospital.

from hospital' care packages providing medical therapy and daily nursing support at home rather than admitting the patient. These are well-liked by the patients, safe and have been shown in two randomized trials to be associated with similar subsequent re-admission rates to conventional therapy. The entry criteria to one of these studies and the home care package are shown in Table 9.3. Earlier discharge from hospital with additional home support is also practical in the two-thirds of cases who still need admitting.

Bronchodilators

At home, the usual bronchodilators can be given more frequently, or bronchodilator therapy initiated for a period in those who are not normally symptomatic. If beta-agonists are used alone, an anticholinergic agent should be added and the dose of both increased to higher levels. A spacer device

should be provided if there is difficulty with inhaler technique.

In hospital, nebulized bronchodilators are the rule, given in high doses. Normally 5 mg of salbutamol and/or 500 µg of ipratropium bromide are used, although some patients are intolerant of the salbutamol owing to tremor and tachycardia. Whether both are needed is contentious. Trials using FEV_1 as the outcome show little difference between the combination and its component parts. The FEV_1 may not be the most sensitive measure in severe disease, however, and many clinicians continue to use both drugs, at least in the early stages of the admission.

Oral corticosteroids

Although seldom used in the UK in mild disease, there is now clear evidence that corticosteroids increase the rate of resolution of more severe exacerbations and shorten hospitalization (Fig. 9.2). Although high doses

Table 9.3
Entry criteria for home care package rather than admission in an exacerbation of COPD.

Patients eligible if:	Patients ineligible if:
$pH > 7.35$	Chest X-ray abnormal
$PaO_2 > 7.3\,kPa$	ECG shows acute change suggestive of
$PaCO_2 < 8.0\,kPa$	ischemia/pulmonary embolus
Heart rate < 100 beats/min	Confused or impaired consciousness
White blood count $4–20 \times 10^9/l$	Requires intravenous therapy
	Needs full time nursing care

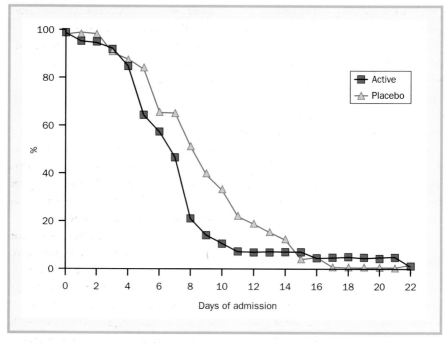

Figure 9.2
Corticosteroid treatment significantly reduces the duration of hospital stay compared with patients on placebo. Modified with permission from Davies et al.[8]

are commonly used in the USA,[7] equivalent results can be achieved using 30 mg per day taken as a single dose for 10 days.[8] Whether these courses can be shortened further and still be beneficial is unknown but it appears possible from the current data. Given the undesirable effects of regular oral therapy, it is essential to definitely stop this treatment at the end of the course. Complex tapering down regimes are normally not needed unless the

patient has had a previous course of treatment in the last few months.

Antibiotics

These are indicated in patients with increased volumes of green sputum — especially if there have been previous upper respiratory tract symptoms.[3] The choice of agent is greatly dependent on local patterns of antibiotic resistance but should cover the major pathogens known to cause exacerbations (see Chapter 7). The impact of this treatment on the course of the disease is surprisingly small but favourable, thus their use can be justified. There is no evidence, however, that more expensive 'modern' antibiotics such as the quinolones or oral cephalosporins are superior to older agents in this condition. Parenteral therapy even in hospital is only indicated when the patient is unable to swallow, since the bioavailability of the usual agents is excellent. Patients with co-existing bronchiectasis are an exception to this rule.

Oxygen

Controlled oxygen therapy sufficient to increase the PaO_2 above 8.0 kPa without inducing or worsening CO_2 retention or respiratory acidosis is the goal of oxygen therapy. This requires selection of an appropriate delivery system and monitoring of the arterial blood gases after therapy begins (approximately 30 minutes after a change in FiO_2 is optimum). Ideally a Venturi® mask device should be used and either 28% or 24% inspired oxygen prescribed. Some patients are very intolerant of this therapy, however, and repeatedly dislodge the mask. Nasal prongs give a less precise inspired oxygen because of associated mouth breathing but are easier for the patient to keep on and allow them to eat and drink while using oxygen. A flow of 2 l/min delivers

approximately 30% oxygen and 1 l/min around 25%. Blood gas monitoring is necessary when this system is used and is needed whenever the $PaCO_2$ is increased. Reliance on pulse oximetry can be dangerously misleading in this setting.

Ventilatory stimulants

Originally used together with physiotherapy to rouse the patient drowsy from CO_2 narcosis and aid secretion clearance, neither physiotherapy or respiratory stimulant drugs are recommended in the management of respiratory failure in COPD. In the former case, there is no evidence that physiotherapy improves blood gas tensions, while concerns about precipitating respiratory muscle fatigue led to the latter treatment being abandoned. This may be unfair since some series suggest that using doxapram intravenously can reduce arterial CO_2 secondary to its non-specific central stimulant effect on breathing. At present this is used to 'buy time' in units where access to other forms of ventilatory support is limited. Intravenous aminophylline is sometimes advocated and often administered as a 'ventilatory stimulant' and non-specific bronchodilator. The evidence to support this practice is non-existent.

Assisted ventilation

This should be considered whenever respiratory acidosis is progressive, despite the therapy already discussed or when acidosis is persistent and the patient is becoming exhausted. General physicians and many pulmonary specialists in the UK have taken an unduly pessimistic view about what this therapy can achieve, which has led to a self-fulfilling prophesy whereby all such patients die and are therefore too sick to be saved. Recent developments in non-invasive ventilatory support may change this.

Non-invasive ventilation

This is accomplished using a full-face mask or nasal mask attached to the patient by adjustable head straps and to a patient-triggered ventilator. Although volume-cycled devices were used initially, most units now use bi-level pressure machines where the level of inspiratory pressure support and continuous positive expiratory pressure can be adjusted independently. The latter is usually set at 5 cm H_2O to counterbalance the increased PEEPi discussed earlier, while the pressure support is increased to the maximum the patient can tolerate, commonly around 15 cm H_2O. The machine passively undertakes part of the work of breathing for the patient and unloads the respiratory muscles. As a result, dyspnoea is lessened and a more mechanically favourable breathing pattern adopted. Clinical studies have shown that this therapy:

• Reduces mortality compared with conventional therapy, at least in patients with a pH under 7.25;[9]

• Reduces hospital stay and the need for intubation/intermittent positive pressure ventilation (IPPV);[10]

• Can be applied in a district general hospital provided simple instructions are provided for the nursing team to follow;

• Increases total nurse contact with the patient by approximately 90 minutes per admission.

The major advantage of this technique is that it avoids the risks of ventilator-associated pneumonia, which is a major hazard of IPPV in these patients. IPPV is not suitable for all cases, however; the following are relative contraindications:

• Confusion;

• Production of excessive amounts of sputum;

• Multisystem failure;

• pH over 7.25;

• Lobar pneumonia.

Intermittent positive pressure ventilation (IPPV)

A full discussion of this is beyond the scope of this book. Mortality as an inpatient from patients going to IPPV is between 15–30% depending on the series and the selection criteria (Table 9.4). Duration of stay in the intensive care unit is longer than average in COPD cases but complete ventilator-

Table 9.4
Principal deciding factors for use of ventilatory support in chronic obstructive pulmonary disease.

Factors to encourage use of IPPV
- *A demonstrable remedial reason for current decline — for example, radiographic evidence of pneumonia or drug overdosage;*
- *The first episode of respiratory failure;*
- *An acceptable quality of life or habitual level of activity.*

Factors likely to discourage use of IPPV
- *Previously documented severe COPD that has been fully assessed and found to be unresponsive to relevant therapy;*
- *A poor quality of life — for example, being housebound, in spite of maximal appropriate therapy;*
- *Severe co-morbidities — for example, pulmonary oedema or neoplasma.*

N.B. Neither age alone nor the PaCO$_2$ are a good guide to the outcome of assisted ventilation in hypercapnic respiratory failure due to COPD. A pH of > 7.26 is a better predictor of survival during the acute episode.

dependence is unusual in the UK. Major complications are listed in Table 9.5.

Successful weaning depends on the underlying severity of the COPD, the extent of intensive care unit-related complications — particularly skeletal muscle myopathy and the patient's nutritional state. Weaning can often be aided by using non-invasive positive pressure ventilation (NIPPV) as a step down approach, although this is difficult in those who have undergone tracheostomy.

Whatever type of therapy is adopted there are clearly cases where use of ventilatory support of any kind is inappropriate. The principal factors relevant to this decision are listed in Table 9.4. Decisions about whether or not to proceed with this therapy should not be left to the most junior or inexperienced member of the medical team, nor should they be based on hearsay or partial information. If there is doubt then it is better to offer the patient the benefit rather than letting a remediable condition prove fatal. The fact

Table 9.5
Complications of intermittent positive pressure ventilation.

Barotrauma (pneumothorax, pneumomediastinum)
Cardiac arrhythmias (atrial tachycardia, atrial fibrillation most often)
Gastrointestinal bleeding
Pulmonary emboli (hard to diagnose)
Nosocomial pneumonia

that this clinical scenario arises at a time when intensive care/medical teams are often at their most stretched does not justify following a path that is easier for the doctors but fatal for the patient.

Patients and their relatives are now more aware of the possible therapies available than previously and it is important that both know when, in the doctor's view, it is no longer appropriate to consider this type of treatment. The development of advanced directives or 'living wills' is potentially time-consuming but important part of modern medical care.

Practical aspects and prevention

The decision to consider discharge is made as much on the general appearance of the patient as on any objective measurement and is often dictated by the availability of carers at home and on social support services. The following steps are always important:

- Stop nebulized bronchodilators 24 hours or more before discharge and substitute with maintenance inhaled bronchodilators;
- Ensure the patient has good inhaler technique and understands how the therapy is to be taken, when to take it and what to do if it stops being effective;
- Arrange outpatient review, especially if domiciliary oxygen is being considered;
- Be clear about when the oral corticosteroid

course ends — consider adding inhaled corticosteroids;
- Assess the social situation — who will cook and shop? Where is the toilet and can it be accessed? How socially isolated is the patient and can this be improved?
- Notify the GP and ensure that he or she knows what the discharge medication is and any important decisions made about future therapy.

Preventing further exacerbations is difficult and the data are confusing. Several drugs have been thought to be effective including:

- Regular or long-acting bronchodilators;
- Inhaled corticosteroids (see Chapter 8);
- Mucolytic agents — particularly *N*-acetyl cysteine. This drug is not licensed in the UK but seems to reduce the number of episodes of chronic bronchitis, mainly in patients with mild COPD;
- OM-BV — this is an 'immunostimulant drug that seems to reduce the severity but not the number of exacerbations according to one well-conducted trial;
- Vaccination – see Chapter 7.

Practical points

- Exacerbations are defined on the basis of a change in symptoms;
- Exacerbations are one of the major drivers of health care costs in COPD;

- Most exacerbations are precipitated by infection but atmospheric pollution and climate changes are also precipitants;
- Exacerbations involve airway narrowing and hyperinflation;
- Home from hospital and rapid discharge teams can shorten or avoid hospital admissions;
- Increased bronchodilator treatment is a mainstay of exacerbation management;
- Oral corticosteroids have proven benefit in severe exacerbations;
- Oxygen is an important treatment but can induce hypercapnia;
- Oxygen saturation alone is inadequate to monitor oxygen therapy;
- Intermittent positive pressure ventilation reduces mortality, length of stay and intubation rates in severe exacerbations with acidosis and hypercapnia.

References

1   Calverley PMA, Rennard S, Agusti AGN, et al. Current and future management of acute exacerbations of chronic obstructive pulmonary disease. *Eur Respir Rev* 1999;9:193–205.

2   Bhowmik A, Seemungal TA, Sapsford RJ, et al. Relation of sputum inflammatory markers to symptoms and exacerbations. *Thorax* 2000;55:114–20.

3   Anthonisen NR, Manfreda J, Warren CP, et al. Antibiotic therapy in exacerbations of chronic obstructive pulmonary disease. *Ann Int Med* 1987;106:196–204.

4   Bhowmik A, Seemungal TA, Sapsford RJ, et al. Comparison of spontaneous and induced sputum for investigation of airway inflammation in chronic obstructive pulmonary disease. *Thorax* 1998;53:953–6.

5   Seemungal TA, Donaldson GC, Paul EA, et al. Effect of exacerbations on quality of life in patients with chronic obstructive pulmonary disease. *Am J Respir Crit Care Med* 1998;157:1418–22.

6   Plant PK, Owen JL, Elliott MW. One year period prevalence study of respiratory acidosis in acute exacerbations of COPD: implications for the provision of non-invasive ventilation and oxygen administration. *Thorax* 2000;55:550–4.

7   Niewoehner DE, Erbland ML, Deupree RH, et al. Effect of systemic glucocorticoids on exacerbations of chronic obstructive pulmonary disease. *New Engl J Med* 1999;340:1941–7.

8   Davies L, Angus RM, Calverley PMA. Oral corticosteroids in patients admitted to hospital with exacerbations of chronic obstructive pulmonary disease: A prospective randomised controlled trial. *Lancet* 1999;354:456–60.

9   Bott J, Carroll MP, Conway JH, et al. Randomised controlled trial of nasal ventilation in acute ventilatory failure due to chronic obstructive airways disease. *Lancet* 1993;341:1555–7.

10 Brochard L, Mancebo J, Wysocki M, et al. Noninvasive ventilation for acute exacerbations of chronic obstructive pulmonary disease. *New Engl J Med* 1995;333:817–22.

Treating the complications of COPD

10

Introduction

As the disease progresses several complications arise beyond those directly related to the disordered lung mechanics that characterize this illness. There is increasing evidence for several 'systemic' problems arising from continuing airway and pulmonary inflammation; these are discussed in Chapter 11, where rehabilitation is considered. This chapter will review briefly the mechanical complications of COPD but most attention will be directed to the problems that arise as a result of hypoxaemia and hypercapnia, the therapy of which is well-defined.

Mechanical problems

Cough syncope

This occurs when the intrathoracic pressure rises abruptly during a bout of coughing and venous return to the right heart is reduced transiently, with a corresponding fall in cardiac output. This is a further example of the problems of dynamic hyperinflation when the next inspiration in the sequence of coughs occurs before expiration is complete and end-expiratory lung volumes increased. There is no evidence-based therapy for this problem but use of a short-acting bronchodilator will help suppress the symptom. The patient should be advised to do an end inspiratory breath-hold, partly to try to delay the next cough but also to allow a slower expiration and thereby reduce the risk of syncope.

Cough fractures

These occur by a similar mechanism to cough syncope, with a vigorous isometric muscle contraction leading to a painful partial or complete fracture in a patient with severe COPD and chronic hyperinflation. Background osteoporosis and oral corticosteroid therapy is usual. Although the ribs are the commonest site of the problems, some patients can precipitate crush fractures of the vertebral bodies in this way.

Spontaneous pneumothorax

This can arise in association with rib fractures but is more often related to subpleural emphysematous change. In general, it is commoner in more severe disease and should always be managed actively. Very small pneumothoraces (less than 15% of the lung) can be observed for spontaneous resolution. If there are increased symptoms or if there is up to 30% deflation, aspiration and observation may be appropriate. Larger pneumothoraces

require formal underwater seal drainage, with an intercostal drain in place until there is complete resolution. In many cases where the underlying emphysema is advanced, a bronchopleural fistula develops and complete re-expansion is not possible. In these circumstances, an early resort to thoracic surgical intervention with video-assisted sealing of the leak and pleurectomy should be made. Patients with two or more uncomplicated pneumothoraces on the same side should also receive this treatment electively.

Chronic respiratory failure

As the mechanical abnormalities that characterize COPD progress, it becomes increasingly difficult to maintain the arterial blood gas tensions within the normal range. Although not studied in a single group of patients, cross-sectional data suggest that failure to maintain oxygenation during exercise is the earliest abnormality followed by the development of clinically significant resting hypoxaemia. This has little impact on exercise performance in its own right since oxygen delivery to exercising muscle depends on the combined effects of the haemoglobin concentration, arterial oxygen saturation of the haemoglobin and cardiac output. The sigmoid shape of the oxygen desaturation curve (ODC) means that saturation does not fall linearly with a decrease in PaO_2 but only changes substantially when the PaO_2 is less than 8.0 kPa. This threshold is used to determine the onset of respiratory failure. Indeed, once oxygen tensions fall to this level at rest when breathing air, important secondary changes develop in the pulmonary circulation and heart, which have a prognostic effect on COPD that is independent of the mechanical abnormality as measured by the predicted FEV_1 percentage. Some of these changes are more likely in patients who develop hypercapnia chronically ($PaCO_2 >$ 6.0 kPa) in whom retention of bicarbonate by renal mechanisms results in a compensated respiratory acidosis.

When these abnormal blood gas tensions are sustained for long periods of time, in other words when the patient is clinically stable but hypoxaemic, three serious but related complications may develop:

1. Pulmonary hypertension;
2. Cor pulmonale;
3. Secondary polycythaemia.

Overall mortality is increased in hypoxaemic COPD that is independent of the severity of airflow limitation, largely because of these complications.

The airways is present in small pulmonary arterioles before the development of respiratory failure, clinically important changes in the physiology of the pulmonary circulation only occur when daytime hypoxaemia is established. Even in severe disease, the resting pulmonary artery pressures are only modestly raised (mean values 35 mmHg) but exercise can produce similar increases in much earlier disease, and pulmonary artery pressures can approach systemic values in severe disease even during the brief periods of exercise that can be sustained. This contributes to exercise limitation, worsens $\dot{V}/Q$ matching and can cause secondary right ventricular hypertrophy. Pulmonary artery pressure is increased during exacerbations but falls to its customary value slowly as the patient recovers. It increases further when the PaO_2 falls during the physiological hypoventilation that accompanies sleep. This may be the earliest stage in the development of daytime pulmonary hypertension but this has not been shown conclusively. Pulmonary hypertension is a predictor of mortality in severe COPD but whether it is superior to the arterial oxygen tension is debatable, thus its routine measurement is not recommended.

Pulmonary hypertension

Although recent data suggest that an inflammatory infiltrate similar to that seen in

Cor pulmonale

This is a pathological term that describes the increased thickness of the right ventricular wall and septum and increased weight of these tissues relative to the left ventricle. It is difficult to interpret these changes when left ventricular disease is present (a common co-morbidity in COPD) since they may occur secondary to left heart failure. This diagnosis is a pathological one and attempts to confirm it in vivo with magnetic resonance imaging (MRI) have proven disappointing. The development of fluid retention (ankle swelling and an increased jugular venous pressure) is often used to infer this condition or at least right heart failure. This is probably incorrect since fluid retention in these patients is associated with reduced right ventricular function and altered renal sodium handling acutely and is normally confined to hypercapnic patients. Right ventricular function returns to normal when the fluid retention resolves or becomes chronic, suggesting that factors other than structural cardiac changes are causing this problem.

Secondary polycythaemia

This is a less frequent complication that is often associated with an increase in facial colouring and an increased haemoglobin value beyond the normal range. The most reliable simple measurement is an increased packed cell volume (PCV) — over 52% in men or to 47% in women. The increased number of red cells and secondary changes in plasma volume alter the rheological properties of the blood,

impairing circulation in the capillary beds of many tissues and promoting venous thrombosis. Although hypoxaemia is necessary for this problem to occur, the most important co-factor is cigarette smoking.[1] Most of the variation in PCV between hypoxaemic COPD patients is explained by the increased levels of carboxyhaemoglobin generated from cigarettes, which provides a further stimulus to red cell production, probably by increasing tissue hypoxaemia in the renal medulla.

Oxygen therapy

This is the most appropriate treatment for each of the complications associated with respiratory failure. Since they arise from conditions of *sustained* hypoxaemia, this therapy should be given for at least 15 hours per day including the sleeping period when oxygen tensions are lowest. Two seminal randomized controlled trials[2,3] showed that this can improve mortality in patients with a PaO_2 of less than 7.3 kPa, prevent the progression of resting pulmonary hypertension, improve neurocognitive function, health status and reduce secondary polycythaemia (Fig. 10.1). In general, the longer the treatment was used through the day the better the survival. Retrospective pathological data suggest that some of the cardiac changes may regress with oxygen therapy. Data about the effects of smoking cessation in these groups are sparse but

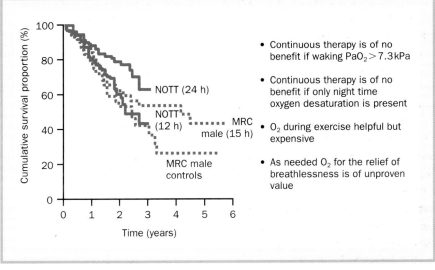

Figure 10.1
Oxygen therapy in chronic obstructive pulmonary disease (COPD). The left-hand panel shows survival experience of patients with stable hypoxaemic COPD and indicates that increased exposure to supplementary oxygen throughout the day prolongs life. The right-hand panel indicates limitations of oxygen treatment in clinical practice. Solid lines = data reproduced from reference 2, dotted lines = data reproduced from reference 3.

strenuous efforts to persuade patients to stop smoking should be made, not least for safety reasons (deaths from smoking while using oxygen have been recorded) but also because this is an important way of improving secondary poycythaemia and continued smoking can block these beneficial effects of oxygen.

Indications

Domiciliary oxygen therapy for more than 15 hours daily is indicated in patients with a spirometrically confirmed diagnosis of COPD and a PaO_2 less than 7.3 kPa when clinically stable. Hypercapnia is not required for treatment to be helpful nor is a history of previous ankle swelling, although both are strong pointers to the need for treatment. Oxygen therapy should not be prescribed:

- If the PaO_2 is in the range 7.3–8.5 kPa, which some have considered an indication previously;

- For isolated nocturnal oxygen desaturation without daytime hypoxaemia;

- When the patient is recovering from an acute exacerbation (some very hypoxaemic patients may be sent home on this therapy but *must* be reviewed to confirm its continued appropriateness).

Practical aspects

Oxygen is an expensive and relatively cumbersome therapy. It can be provided in three ways:

1. Oxygen concentrators: these are static units where a xeolite membrane separates oxygen from room air. Fixed units consume domestic electricity (usually re-imbursed in the UK). Lengths of plastic tubing permit use around the house but not beyond. Home maintenance and servicing is provided by independent contractors in the UK. This is by far the most economic way of providing oxygen for use more than 5 hours per day. Portable units have been developed but remain experimental and heavy.
2. Liquid oxygen: this method is widely used in the USA but is very expensive. A reservoir tank is filled regularly by the supplier and smaller portable unit can be filled at home to permit oxygen therapy when walking (see later text).
3. Cylinder oxygen: this is a cumbersome and relatively expensive method of long-term oxygen administration. In the UK, it is

provided by oxygen-dispensing pharmacists. There is a significant rental charge for the cylinder irrespective of the gas within it (see later text), and cylinder oxygen is difficult for the patient to handle but it is widely available.

Oxygen can be given either by Venturi mask (controlled flow at a fixed percentage of gas) or by nasal prongs at a specified flow rate (1–3 l/min). The choice will depend on patient preference and, in each case, the flow rate/concentration should be specified based on the response to oxygen therapy in the laboratory. Effective therapy must increase the PaO_2 to over 8.0 kPa. Worsening of CO_2 retention in these stable patients is surprisingly uncommon even at higher flow rates of oxygen.

Oxygen-conserving devices, which range from simple plastic reservoirs that collect gas to more technical timing mechanisms that deliver oxygen only during inspiration, can increase the time before exhaustion of portable oxygen cylinders (which usually last 30–60 minutes) and hence permit outdoor exercise for some patients. These devices can have economic advantages if liquid systems are used but have not been adopted in the UK. Transtracheal oxygen cuts down upper airway dead space and permits adequate oxygenation at lower flow rates; however problems with local bleeding and blockage of the mini-tracheostomy needed for this treatment have prevented its widespread acceptance.

Other uses of oxygen therapy

Increasing exercise capacity

Use of oxygen during exercise increases the distance walked and, more dramatically, the *duration* of exercise, while reducing the intensity of dyspnoea (probably by decreasing minute ventilation at any work intensity). These effects are best seen in hypoxaemic patients but also occur when the PaO_2 is relatively preserved. The benefits of portable oxygen are lost if the patient has to carry the weight of the oxygen cylinder so a wheeled carrier should be provided. Continued smoking further limits the improvement in exercise capacity.[4] Selection of patients is often based on the resting PaO_2 and/or the presence of desaturation during exercise, although this has never been tested formally to confirm its usefulness as a selection criterion. The benefits of ambulatory oxygen are modest and it is not widely prescribed in the UK. This may restrict the mobility of these disabled patients even more.

Short-term relief of breathlessness

This is one of the commonest uses of cylinder oxygen, at least in the UK. It is relatively expensive, poorly regulated and its benefits are based on very limited information. How much of these are a placebo effect and how much physiological is unknown, although a few studies suggest that dyspnoea can be reduced by treatment with oxygen before or after exercise.

Other therapies

Pulmonary vasodilators

A range of smooth muscle relaxant drugs including hydralazine have been used to treat pulmonary hypertension in COPD with little success. Nitric oxide at rest worsens blood gas tensions despite being the most specific pulmonary vasodilator known. Almitrine bismethylate modifies local pulmonary vasoconstriction and is a specific peripheral chemoreceptor stimulant that can increase resting PaO_2. It can precipitate peripheral neuropathy, however, and is not widely licensed for use in COPD.

Venesection

Venesection is still used in patients with severe polycythaemia who do not respond to oxygen therapy. Removal of a unit of blood with replacement with an equivalent volume of dextran produces variable improvement in exercise performance and reductions in headache. The duration of this benefit is extremely variable.

Chronic ventilatory support

This is still an experimental approach to therapy, which is largely confined to the oxygen-intolerant patients with significant daytime hypoxaemia and hypercapnia. Contrary to early expectations, respiratory support with negative or nasal positive pressure ventilation did not change the symptoms or prognosis of normocapnic COPD patients. Hypercapnic COPD patients treated with night-time nasal ventilation and domiciliary oxygen felt better and had better blood gas concentrations than those treated with oxygen alone, and uncontrolled case series suggest they may also have a survival benefit. Nevertheless, this treatment should be restricted to highly selected cases in experienced treatment centres until more data are available.

The 'overlap syndrome'

This inelegant term refers to the co-existence of COPD and obstructive sleep apnoea, something that occurs by chance infrequently since both are relatively prevalent conditions. It is usually diagnosed when the patient develops a clinical picture of acute fluid retention similar to cor pulmonale but has an FEV_1 of over 1.5 l and/or a PaO_2 of 8.0 kPa. The repetitive nocturnal hypoxaemia associated with sleep apnoea is the trigger to this and appropriate history-taking will usually reveal the cardinal clinical features of this condition — snoring and daytime somnolence. Treatment is with nasal continuous positive pressure, although patients with waking hypoxaemia may need supplementary oxygen overnight. Effective therapy of the sleep apnoea can cause a

reduction in waking hypoxaemia even in COPD, probably by a resetting of the chemoreceptor gain.

Practical points

- Syncope, rib fractures and pneumothorax are possible complications of coughing in severe COPD;

- Pulmonary hypertension and cor pulmonale are complications of hypoxia in COPD;

- Long-term home oxygen therapy improves mortality in hypoxaemic COPD patients;

- Criteria for use of long-term oxygen therapy require arterial blood gas analysis;

- Oxygen concentrators are the most economical way to deliver oxygen for more than 5 hours per day;

- In long-term oxygen therapy oxygen should be used for as many hours a day as possible, with 15 hours as a minimum;

- Occasional use of oxygen from cylinders may be of minor benefit for symptom relief in some patients;

- The 'overlap syndrome' of COPD and obstructive sleep apnoea should be considered in patients with daytime somnolence or cor pulmonale without profound hypoxia;

- Occasional patients may benefit from non-invasive ventilation at home.

References

1   Calverley PM, Leggett RJ, McElderry L, Flenley DC. Cigarette smoking and secondary polycythemia in hypoxic cor pulmonale. *Am Rev Respir Dis* 1982;**125**:507–10.

2   Anonymous. Continuous or nocturnal oxygen therapy in hypoxemic chronic obstructive lung disease: a clinical trial. Nocturnal Oxygen Therapy Trial Group. *Ann Int Med* 1980;**93**:391–8.

3   Anonymous. Long term domiciliary oxygen therapy in chronic hypoxic cor pulmonale complicating chronic bronchitis and emphysema. Report of the Medical Research Council Working Party. *Lancet* 1981;**1**:681–6.

4   Calverley PM, Leggett RJ, Flenley DC. Carbon monoxide and exercise tolerance in chronic bronchitis and emphysema. *Brit Med J Clin Res* 1981;**283**:878–80.

Lifestyle modification

11

Introduction

In this chapter some of the other therapeutic approaches to COPD will be reviewed. The most important change in lifestyle any COPD patient can make is to quit smoking. This has been reviewed in Chapter 4. Two other useful approaches are related to exercise and appropriate nutrition, which form important parts of the process of pulmonary rehabilitation. This is dealt with in detail, since it is an underused treatment approach that offers real benefits to patients at all stages of COPD and is complementary to pharmacological treatment approaches. Finally, some of the actions that should be taken by the patient to recognize and monitor their progress will be reviewed.

Pulmonary rehabilitation

Patients with COPD, particularly those with moderate to severe symptoms, experience a range of non-pulmonary problems including:

- Exercise de-conditioning;
- Relative social isolation;

- Altered mood states, especially depression;
- Muscle wasting and weight loss.

These problems have complex interrelationships. Thus a high total energy expenditure contributes to weight loss but circulating inflammatory markers may further promote specific muscle pathology. In approximately one-third of patients, dyspnoea alone limits exercise performance; in another one-third tiredness is the limiting factor; the remaining one-third of patients report equivalent limitation by both symptoms.[1]

While dyspnoea results primarily from intrinsic lung disease, its perceived magnitude is influenced by mental state, which is also a major determinant of exercise performance and under self-paced conditions in COPD. Improvement in any one of these interlinked processes can promote a 'virtuous spiral', where positive gains occur in all aspects of the illness (Fig. 11.1). Pulmonary rehabilitation is a process whereby many of these extra-pulmonary problems can be addressed.

No universally agreed definition of pulmonary rehabilitation exists but that

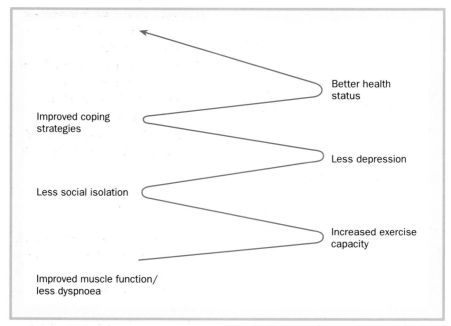

Figure 11.1
The 'virtuous spiral' of pulmonary rehabilitation.

recommended by the American Thoracic Society incorporates most of the essential features:

'Pulmonary rehabilitation is a multidisciplinary programme of care for patients with chronic respiratory impairment that is individually tailored and designed to optimize physical and social performance'

Key elements within this process include:

- Assessments of the total impact of the disease on the individual, their lifestyle and family;
- Patient education;
- The role of exercise, nutrition and oxygen treatment;
- The development of an individual treatment plan and the identification of the individual's need for psychological and social support at home.

Initial enthusiasm for pulmonary rehabilitation waned when it failed to change measurements of lung mechanics. There is now clear evidence that treatment is beneficial and this will be reviewed before examining the components of the programme itself.

Evidence of benefit

Pulmonary rehabilitation has been evaluated carefully in many clinical trials comprising both open and randomized controlled studies. Comprehensive reviews of these data now exist, itemizing individual studies and the benefits demonstrated.[2] Moreover specific meta-analysis of the available randomized clinical trials has been conducted.[3] These reviews allow the following statements to be made:

1. There is strong evidence from randomized controlled clinical trials that pulmonary rehabilitation improves exercise capacity, reduces the intensity of perceived breathlessness, reduces the number of hospitalizations and days in hospital and has benefits that extend well beyond the immediate period of training.[4]
2. There is observational evidence and some clinical data to support the view that pulmonary rehabilitation that includes strength and endurance training of the upper limbs improves arm function and can improve health-related quality of life.

Expert opinion and more limited data supports the views that:

- Respiratory muscle training is beneficial in COPD — especially when combined with general exercise training;
- Psychosocial intervention is helpful in COPD;
- Pulmonary rehabilitation may improve survival.

Components of the programme

Education

Most programmes include specific information about the nature of COPD, how to optimize medical treatment, including inhaler technique, general information about nutrition and breathing exercises. Specific techniques for the latter have been advocated but when evaluated have not always proven to be well based scientifically. This is particularly true for diaphragmatic breathing, which is associated with increased respiratory muscle work. Objective evidence to support use of an educational package as a sole strategy in rehabilitation is lacking. It is not yet clear whether inclusion of the educational component is necessary for those undergoing exercise training to obtain maximum benefit.

Exercise

A range of exercise strategies have been employed — with home cycle ergometry and treadmill walking being the most studied. Exercise frequency ranges from daily to weekly, its duration from 10 minutes to 45 minutes per session, its intensity from 50% $\dot{V}O_{2\,max}$ to maximum tolerated. Programmes vary from 4–46 weeks in duration with most being 8–10 weeks long. General exercise guidelines are given in Table 11.1. Intensity is usually monitored by trying to obtain a pre-set target heart rate but this may not be the

Table 11.1
General exercise guidelines in chronic obstructive pulmonary disease.

Patients should exercise:
– *for at least 20 minutes continuously*
– *for at least 3 sessions per week (2 supervised)*
– *until they become uncomfortably breathless*
– *to the same level of symptoms in each session*
– *using corridor walking, treadmill or cycle exercise*
– *according to an individualized plan*

most appropriate measure in COPD. Many programmes, especially those using simple corridor exercise training encourage the patient to walk to a symptom-limited maximum, rest and continue walking until 20 minutes of exercise has been completed.

Upper limb exercises

This is usually achieved by use of an upper limb ergometer or resistive training with weights. There are no randomized clinical trial data to support its routine use, but it may be helpful in those with co-morbidities which restrict other forms of exercise.

Nutrition

See separate section.

Psychological well-being

Depression and anxiety are frequent findings in COPD and merit specific reassurance and where appropriate, medical treatment, although dependence on anxiolytic drugs is to be avoided. Oral corticosteroids promote depression and more seriously proximal muscle myopathy and should be withdrawn if at all possible. Pulmonary rehabilitation programmes can produce non-specific improvements in both anxiety and depression scores for reasons that are not entirely clear. Likewise specific programmes directed at controlling breathlessness have met with variable success; this may reflect the relative enthusiasm of the therapists involved.

Patient assessment

This should include:

- A detailed history and physical examination;
- A measurement of spirometry before and after bronchodilator drug;
- An assessment of exercise capacity;
- A measurement of the impact of breathlessness and/or health status.

Other physiological tests might include an assessment of inspiratory and expiratory muscle strength and lower limb strength, for example quadriceps in cases where muscle wasting is important.

Exercise capacity can be quantified using progressive or treadmill exercise testing, with ventilatory recordings including oxygen consumption and minute ventilation together with blood lactate. Simpler tests such as self-paced timed walking tests appear to give reliable if less-complete information, provided care is taken to familiarize the patient with at least two practice walks before the initial assessment. The shuttle walking tests offer a compromise between maximum and entirely self-paced test while remaining relatively simple to perform. Recording of the intensity of breathlessness before and at the end of exercise using either a visual analogue scale or a modified Borg scale increases the utility of testing.

The impact of breathlessness on daily activities can be assessed simply using the modified Medical Research Council scale or the baseline dyspnoea index, which is more sensitive to changes following an intervention when it is combined with the transitional dyspnoea index. Some have suggested that stratification by breathlessness intensity using the MRC questionnaire may be helpful in selecting patients most likely to benefit from rehabilitation.[5]

Health status sometimes termed 'quality of life', can be assessed either in general terms using the Modified Short Form 36 Questionnaire, or more specifically related to respiratory functions using the Chronic Respiratory Questionnaire or the St George's

Respiratory Questionnaire — both of which give reproducible and validated information about the impact of COPD on health. Although widely translated, they may not always be accessible in an appropriate local language and are relatively time-consuming to complete. A shorter 20-question version is being developed, which may prove applicable to routine clinical care.

Patient selection

More information is needed about those patients most likely to benefit. Early worries that only those able to exceed the anaerobic threshold would benefit have proven groundless. Benefits have also been seen in a wide range of disability, although patients who are chair-bound appear unlikely to respond even to home-visiting programmes. The most important considerations in choosing patients are:

* Motivation: especially if outpatient programmes are employed;
* Co-morbidities: exercise performance that is limited by cardiovascular or muscular skeletal disorders is less likely to improve in a rehabilitation setting.

Setting

Benefits have been reported in inpatient, outpatient and home programmes.

Considerations of cost and availability will determine the choice but indirect evidence suggests that improvement in the most severe cases, for example in patients on the waiting list for transplantation is most likely with inpatient treatment.

Personnel

Ideally a multi-professional approach should be used with the respiratory therapist taking a lead in the assessment and exercise training but councillors, social workers (if available), nutritionalists and doctors all have a distinctive role. While this is a counsel of perfection, significant benefits can occur when dedicated professionals are aware of the needs of their patient. Optimal group size varies but appears to be best when six or eight individuals are combined in a class.

Follow-up

To date, there is no consensus on whether repeated rehabilitation courses sustain the benefit of the initial assessment; however, it is likely that regimes designed to maintain the level of fitness attained will be worthwhile. The optimum regime to be followed has not been defined. Recent, uncontrolled data suggest that improvements in health status can be protracted even after a single course of treatment.

Nutrition

Obesity can co-exist with severe COPD, increasing the energy required for any amount of exercise and pre-disposing to obstructive sleep apnoea. When this overlap syndrome occurs, fluid retention and cor pulmonale develop at levels of airflow obstruction not usually considered severe. The appropriate treatment is with nasal continuous positive airway pressure at night and a reduced calorie diet.

Many COPD patients appear to be obese but in fact are not since their abdomens are prominent because of pulmonary overinflation. Approximately 25% of patients with moderate-to-severe COPD show a reduction in both their body mass index (BMI) and fat free mass. A reduction in body mass index is an independent risk factor for an increased mortality in COPD, and such patients are less able to undertake activity in the home. Improving the nutritional state of such patients is possible and can lead to improved respiratory muscle strength but there is still controversy as to whether the additional effort is cost-efficient. The results of one large study have suggested that those patients whose BMI improves with nutritional supplementation have a better survival experience. Likewise, there may be some advantage in giving nutritional supplements during an acute exacerbation.[6]

Specific nutritional recommendations are based on expert opinion and some small randomized clinical trials rather than larger studies of the impact of these recommendations routine practice. Key concepts are:

1. The identification of the reasons for reduced calorie intake and their correction:
   - Breathlessness while eating: advise small frequent meals;
   - Poor dentition: correct
   - Co-morbidities such as: pulmonary sepsis, lung tumours etc.: manage as appropriate;
2. Provision of a nutritionally appropriate diet: increased calorie intake improves respiratory muscle strength in the short term but randomized studies suggest that the resulting rise in body mass index is the result of fat deposition rather than an increased muscle mass. Addition of anabolic agents such as the androgens can convert calories to muscle mass but their longer-term use is limited by side-effects. At present, increasing calorie intake is best combined with exercise regimes that have a non-specific anabolic action. This approach has not been tested formally in large numbers of subjects.

Self-management and patient education

In contrast to asthma, there are little data about the effectiveness of self-management plans in COPD. This illness is intrinsically less variable than asthma and so the success of therapy cannot be judged by an improvement in diurnal variability of peak expiratory flow (PEF). The limited data available suggests that PEF only changes in most patients with the onset of an exacerbation and, even then, this is often only a small absolute reduction. Only one report of a specifically designed self management plan is presently available.[7] This was a relatively small study but the authors were able to show that patients who used their plan were better able to manage exacerbations of their disease. More clear-cut improvements in well-being could not, however, be shown. This reflects the slower pace of change in COPD compared with asthma and the need for longer-term and larger studies.

Any self management strategy should focus on:

1. Encouraging abstinence from cigarettes. This may be a small part of the process in a long standing ex-smoker but, even here, noting continued abstinence provides a positive reinforcement to the individual that they have taken action to help themselves. For those who have lapsed but not started to smoke regularly, contact numbers to local support services should be made available as well as a non-threatening approach to helping them quit again.

2. Symptom intensity should be monitored.

At present simple Likert scales, ranging from 'much better than usual' to 'much worse than usual' can give patient and doctor a rapid overview of general progress and signal the start of an exacerbation. Two or more days of 'much worse than usual' should trigger a PEF recording for comparison with the patient's customary value. Key symptoms will normally be cough, sputum production and dyspnoea. It is useful to note the ability to undertake a particular activity relevant to the patient and score the ability to do this.

3. Development of symptoms of an exacerbation should prompt early treatment. This would include an increase in the dose and frequency of bronchodilators, beginning a course of oral corticosteroids and antibiotics if preset thresholds are met. This may prevent hospitalization in some cases.

4. Completion of individual exercise targets: This can be a useful way of monitoring progress, and may sustain the benefits of rehabilitation and help the patient by demonstrating that they can do something to help themselves.

Although this approach sounds rather 'woolly' its rigorous application with regular telephone support has been shown, in Canada, to produce significant reductions in health care contacts and improvement in the patients' health status. Which components of this

Table 11.2
Commonly asked questions that follow a diagnosis of chronic obstructive pulmonary disorder or a recent hospitalization resulting from chronic obstructive pulmonary disorder.

What is COPD?
What causes COPD?
How will it affect me?
Can it be treated?
What should I do if my disease gets worse?
What will happen if I need to be admitted to hospital?
How will I know if I need oxygen at home?
Can I decide when to stop treatment?

approach are most valid remains to be determined. At present, this approach seems most valuable for patients with well-established airflow limitation, that is, an FEV_1 less than 50% predicted.

Patient education alone has relatively little impact on the usual markers of disease control but helps in explaining what they can expect from their illness and improves decision-making about advanced directives. Table 11.2 lists some of the commonly asked questions that follow a diagnosis of COPD or a recent hospitalization due to the disease.

Many patients benefit from participating in some form of self-help group. These groups often start from patients undergoing rehabilitation who want to keep in touch with others who have shared this experience; these people become the nucleus of a local Breathe Easy group. This is the patient's wing of the British Lung Foundation, the principal UK charity concerned with COPD research. The mutual support these meetings offer can be of considerable benefit to a group of patients many of whom feel socially isolated and who are often stigmatized for creating their own illness by smoking. The address for the organizers and some other useful information is listed in the Appendix.

Practical points

- 'Pulmonary rehabilitation is a multidisciplinary program of care for patients with chronic respiratory impairment that is individually tailored and designed to optimize physical and social performance' (ATS);

- Pulmonary rehabilitation improves exercise capacity, reduces breathlessness and reduces hospital admissions and bed days;

- A major part of rehabilitation programmes involves leg exercises through walking or cycling;

- Arm exercises and breathing exercises probably add a little to rehabilitation programmes;

- Rehabilitation programmes usually involve nutritional advice, occupational therapy, social support and education;

- The most important factors in patient selection are motivation and co-morbidities that limit exercise;
- Rehabilitation programmes have been run for inpatients, outpatients or a mixture;
- The optimum regime to maintain the initial benefit is uncertain;
- Nutritional problems of obesity or weight loss are common in COPD.

References

1   Killian KJ, LeBlanc P, Martin DH, et al. Exercise capacity and ventilatory, circulatory, and symptom limitation in patients with chronic airflow limitation. *Am Rev Respir Dis* 1992;**146**:935–40.

2   Ries AL, Carlin BW, Carlin V, et al. Pulmonary rehabilitation: Joint ACCP/AACVPR evidence-based guidelines. *J Cardiopul Rehab* 1997;**17**:371–405.

3   Lacasse Y, Wong E, Guyatt GH, et al. Meta-analysis of respiratory rehabilitation in chronic obstructive pulmonary disease. *Lancet* 1996;**348**:1115–19.

4   Griffiths TL, Burr ML, Campbell IA, et al. Results at 1 year of out-patient multidisciplinary pulmonary rehabilitation. *Lancet* 2000;**355**:362–8.

5   Wedzicha JA, Bestall JC, Garrod R, et al. Randomized controlled trial of pulmonary rehabilitation in severe chronic obstructive pulmonary disease patients, stratified with the MRC dyspnoea scale. *Eur Respir J* 1998;**12**:363–9.

6   Schols AM, Slangen J, Volovics L, Wouters EF. Weight loss is a reversible factor in the prognosis of chronic obsructive pulmonary disease. *Am J Respir Crit Care Med* 1998;**157**:1791–7.

7   Watson PB, Town GI, Holbrook N, et al. Evaluation of a self-management plan for chronic obstructive pulmonary disease. *Eur Respir J* 1997;**10**:1267–71.

Index